SAVING ME FIRST
III

SAVING ME FIRST
III

Unlocking

What's Always Within Us

Hui Beop

Art by Julie Kim

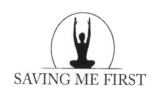

SAVING ME FIRST

Dedication

This book is dedicated to
all who contribute to humanity
and inspire us to learn, to grow,
and to evolve.

And,
to individuals on their journey of self-discovery,
encompassing the wholeness of
mind, body, and spirit.

Contents

Chapter 1   Me and My Organs

Chapter 2   The Nature of Organs

Chapter 3   Organs and Their Symptoms

Chapter 4   Food for the Organs

Chapter 5   DNA

Chapter 6   How to Improve

Chapter 7   External Energies

Chapter 8   More Things We Can Do to Improve

Chapter 9   The Cycle of Seasons

Chapter 1

Me and My Organs

$1,000 Cash Gift and ROI*
*return on the gift

What if we were lucky enough to have been born with a body system that actually distributes power equally among the five organs and is able to occasionally adjust the distribution of that power when the need arises? This would allow the whole system to work much better, freeing us from the daily burden of pain, confusion, and suffering. We would be seeing, knowing, and perceiving in ways that would allow us to easily handle ourselves and others in our everyday lives.

However, most of us aren't that lucky. From time to time, we find ourselves struggling as we work on ourselves physically, mentally, emotionally, and spiritually.

First, let's begin understanding ourselves through a mental exercise. Let's say someone in our family gave us a $1,000 cash gift. Without the filter of learned behavior, such as "we should" or "we shouldn't," observe how we feel. How would we react and how would we decide to fairly repay the kind gesture?

And second, let's invest $1,000 in gifts for our loved ones, family members, friends, workers, etc. without any preconceived notions of what will happen.

We must observe only, without judgments! And we mustn't go around telling people all the things we've discovered about others. Keeping this kind of observation to ourselves is the mature thing to do because this is just for our learning—and we have much more to learn. This is just to know, acknowledge, and to let go with a confirmation, "Ah, so it is."

We might already have some past experience that we can draw from to reflect and recognize certain behaviors. We've made mental notes, but we don't know which of our organ systems played a role in those behaviors. As each organ system has different character traits with different reactions and behaviors, a situation like this often reveals the dominant organ. This is a simple way to understand a very complicated organ system.

We may be thinking that what we feel and express everyday is 100 percent us. But emotions and feelings are part of the organ function. Though it's *part* of us, it's not the *whole* us.

Let's learn the different parts of us through our organs and later understand our whole self. This is a simplified way to determine an organ-type person.

The five major organs are Kidney, Heart, Liver, Lung, and Stomach. These organs have connected organs as well, but for this section, we will discuss only the five major organs. These five organs play very important roles in the functioning of our body system, affecting how we live and die. And each of these organs has a very unique task and set of habits, accompanied by emotions particular to that organ.

How much return we will receive on our investment of $1,000 will be different for each organ type. There is no right or wrong in any of these cases. It is simply for us to know that it is what it is.

Now, we carry out the $1,000 cash gift to our family and friends and observe the corresponding ROI (return on investment).

Strong Kidney

This organ person knows money well and will accept it nicely and keep it, putting it away. It is hard to read this person, but he/she *loves* money and is very selfish when it comes to money. 1/100 return.

Likes: Talking
Dislikes: Anything standing in the way

Strong Heart

This person will accept it with gratitude. For this person, the money is a gift and he/she loves to receive gifts without too many obligations. This person will be thinking about how to spend the money on their next shopping trip. Your return is a bright, happy smile with a kiss on the cheek, a hug, or a well-written thank-you note.

Likes: Shopping
Dislikes: Being without an audience, Confinement

Strong Liver

This person has integrity and modest assets. If he is in need of that gift, he will accept and promise to return 100% of it. The promise will be kept. If this person doesn't need the gift, he/she will reject it. However, if we insist on giving the gift, this person may consider donating it to a good cause. There is no greed and his response is very simple, with kind thoughts of others.

Likes: Reading books and listening to music, etc.
Dislikes: Confinement, Losing face/Being disgraced

Strong Lung

This person likes to earn his/her own way, and doesn't like being indebted or obligated to anyone. This person may refuse the gift. If he/she accepts the gift, the person will find a way to compensate for the gift directly/indirectly now or later in the future. This person will pay back 100% if he/she finds that they need to accept the gift. It will really bother this person not to pay all of it back. No joking!

Likes: Independence
Dislikes: Lies, Injustice, Disorganization

Strong Stomach

This person is an accumulator, and so will take the gift with great appreciation accompanied by sincere words. This person sees everything through money. ROI can be 1/100 of what was given, but with many sweet words of appreciation. The strong Stomach body-type person isn't generous about giving back because his/her body system can't imagine doing more. The body system lacks the fluid for circulation that allows it to give more generously. It always feels like there is never enough as it blindly seeks to fill a perpetual endless need.

Likes: Frugal shopping
Dislikes: Wasting money/resource/things

Determining Your Organ System

Organs and Their Face Shapes

Other clues to identifying an organ type can be found in the face shape and what exclusively moves a person to act. *These are pure organ shapes that do not factor in external energies, or combination of organs.*

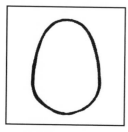

Kidney Type Behavior
Very talkative
Motivated by:
Intellectual Senses

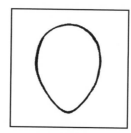

Heart Type Behavior
Loves shopping
Motivated by:
Popularity

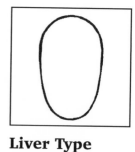

Liver Type Behavior
Likes to read and listen to music
Motivated by:
Integrity and Good Cause

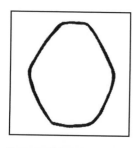

Lung Type Behavior
Independent and likes to direct others
Motivated by:
Principle, What is Right and Just

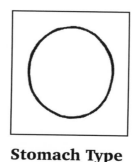

Stomach Type Behavior
Frugal shopper
Motivated by:
Money, Accumulation

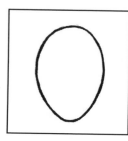

Ideal Shape
Overall harmonized

Besides the general face shape, there are also distinctive facial features that can give clues to the organ type.

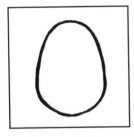

**Kidney Type
Facial Features**
Pronounced chin and muscular lower jaw, with thick healthy hair

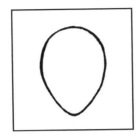

**Heart Type
Facial Features**
Pale dull skin, with pointy chin and shorter distance between nose and upper lip (philtrum)

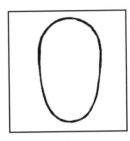

**Liver Type
Facial Features**
Long narrow face, usually has distinct large round eyes, and thick hair

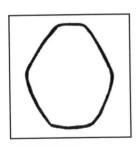

**Lung Type
Facial Features**
Generally has tall handsome nose, naturally good teeth, strong cheek bones, with strong healthy skin

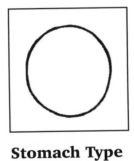

**Stomach Type
Facial Features**
Fullness around lower face and chin area, fleshy cheeks with stocky neck

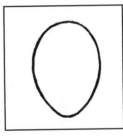

Ideal Shape
Naturally attractive face (without plastic surgery), overall balanced features

Some may have a combination of face shapes and habits, indicating that there are several major organs playing out in us with overlapping traits. The most dominant trait or feature will determine the organ type person.

Behavioral Questionnaire

We sometimes confuse our innate organ traits with behavioral and emotional responses that have been conditioned by our upbringing and our environment. When taking the test, please keep in mind that this is to identify traits that are naturally inherent in your personality, not something learned.

Please answer each question as it best applies to you by circling Y (Yes) or N (No). Giving 10 points for each Y, tally the score at the bottom of each section. For example: 5Y would equal 50 points. If you agree with the statements half way, then you can give it 5 points.

KI

I always tend to underestimate my abilities.	Y	N
In general, I think gloomy and pessimistic thoughts.	Y	N
I am usually uncomfortable being in a group of people.	Y	N
I should probably be less moody and sensitive all the time.	Y	N
In my introspection, I tend to relive past events over and over again.	Y	N
I have a somewhat defensive and touchy nature.	Y	N
I tend to be serious and feel things very deeply.	Y	N
My mind is always thinking up new creations or new ways of doing things.	Y	N
I need to stop worrying all the time.	Y	N
I'm a good researcher.	Y	N

KI Total _____

HE

Socially, I am a pretty outgoing person.	Y	N
I see myself as a cheerful and sociable person.	Y	N
I tend to be a pretty easy-going person.	Y	N
I usually have a good time at parties.	Y	N

I enjoy people and make friends easily.	Y	N
I don't mind simultaneously belonging to several different organizations.	Y	N
In social situations, I am talkative and spontaneous.	Y	N
I like attention and being popular.	Y	N
I like to live my life as freely as possible, without rules and obligations.	Y	N
My friends would describe me as an extrovert.	Y	N

HE Total ____

LI

I seldom get angry or emotional.	Y	N
I have a natural tendency to promote, educate, and mentor people in hopes of improving their lives.	Y	N
I'd like to grow freely, unhampered.	Y	N
I'd like to have vast amounts of knowledge.	Y	N
I am proud and like to be respected.	Y	N
I strongly dislike fighting and inhumane mistreatment of people.	Y	N
It usually takes something drastic to get me excited or upset.	Y	N
I am kind and gentle in spirit.	Y	N
I often have trouble finishing things that I've started.	Y	N
My friends would describe me as an introvert.	Y	N

LI Total ____

LU

A strong will is one my best assets.	Y	N
I almost always finish what I have started, and unfinished projects really bother me.	Y	N

I am self-motivated and always well organized in my work.	Y	N
I have a pretty good ability to get things done.	Y	N
I have strong leadership abilities and consider myself fair-minded.	Y	N
I don't like anything that is disorganized.	Y	N
I tend to work hard and persistently.	Y	N
I can't stand injustice and corruption.	Y	N
I have a fairly keen mind and can usually plan worthwhile long-range projects.	Y	N
I know where I want to go and am usually disciplined enough to get there.	Y	N

LU Total ____

ST

I generally resent those who oppose me.	Y	N
I am good at managing relationships with other people.	Y	N
People often view me as a unifier.	Y	N
I have a habit of remembering all the moments that people have insulted me.	Y	N
I have a tendency to hold grudges against people who were rude to me, and sometimes fantasize about getting revenge for old wrongs.	Y	N
I hate wasting money, and consider myself a frugal shopper.	Y	N
I have a tendency to hold on to old used items "just in case."	Y	N
I have a deep tendency to hold on to money and save it somewhere.	Y	N
I don't trust anyone with my money.	Y	N
I often have negative thoughts.	Y	N

ST Total _____

Please record all the scores on the following Score Summary page.

Score Summary

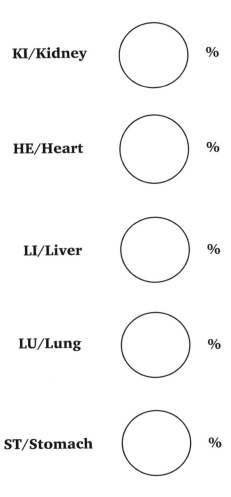

KI/Kidney   %

HE/Heart   %

LI/Liver   %

LU/Lung   %

ST/Stomach   %

60-100 points strong/above normal
50-59 points normal/okay
0-49 points weak/insufficient

Interpreting the scores:

If your score for HE is 60 points or more, and score for LU is 20 points, this means that you should avoid all Heart foods and work toward bringing the Lungs up to Heart score by taking in Lung foods. When you have enough built up, retake the test for the Lung portion. It should show changes. Retake the test every 6 to 12 months to look for changes in results.

What if I found just one organ type that describes me?

It's very simple and easy to recognize. That's the good part. However, having only one dominating strong organ will cause terrible deficiencies in our body system and will become dangerous when we are sick. (*See* "Organs and Their Symptoms," Chapter 3.)

What if I found multiple organ types that describe me?

It's good that we have more than one. It is possible to have one strong organ with 1–3 organs playing more minor roles. It all depends on how our organ systems are powered.

Some people may have multiple traits that come out at the same time or have just one come out if they are all equally powered. This could create some confusion in trying to recognize the dominant organ. (*See* "Organs and Their Symptoms," Chapter 3)

What if the three organs are equally strong?

With three strong organs, let's say that we recognized the traits of strong Heart, strong Stomach, and strong Lungs. That leaves us with our Liver and Kidney systems insufficiently supporting our entire system. To be whole and attain better health, we would need to provide these weaker insufficient energy organs with the foods they need. (*See* "How to Improve My Health," Chapter 6, *see also* the food lists for Liver and Kidney in Chapter 4.)

As we continue our observations, we occasionally find that there are exceptions such as learned traits. This creates confusion when we try to use behavioral patterns to pinpoint the organ type of a person in determining their illness. The learned traits have come about through socialization and survival needs, and they become habits that we mistakenly believe to be our natural original habits. Unfortunately, when one of our organs is sick and we look for traits to identify it, these learned traits ends up getting in the way.

It's very important to understand our body's real feelings, the real emotions that come with each organ. This isn't about making ourselves uncomfortable. Rather, it's about honestly acknowledging what we truly feel and making adjustments when we need to. This is how we take care of ourselves because a strong or a weak organ can break our body system and make it prone to illness.

There are only a very few in the general population who have a harmonized body system, while the vast majority of people are in need of adjustments. We are all in this together as we learn to make a better life for ourselves and others.

Which organ system is better?

We need to respect all of the body's organ systems, as they each serve a unique essential purpose. Ultimately, we must work toward recovering the full function of all our organ systems so that we can finally become whole and fully functioning beings. Until then, we are a work in progress striving to reach that holy state.

What happens if I stay as is and enjoy all the food that strengthens my strong organ?

We will end up following the course of our strong organ's life, habits, and desires. Despite what they may believe, the strong organs need the weaker organs to support them so they can live a better life. Continuing to damage the weaker organs is essentially a death sentence.

When the car battery's juice is spent, that car battery dies. Though we can purchase a new car battery at a store, we can't purchase a new body. This is the only body we'll have in this life.

Once at a wedding, a mother-in-law told her new son-in-law, "Son, please take good care of my daughter. I am too old to make another daughter to take her place if something happens to her."

We must take good care of ourselves through keen observation and fair play when it comes to our body.

How is it going to affect my body if I stay with a strong single organ system?

It depends on how the rest of the organs contribute to the overall system, but it typically follows that the weak or the strong organ will be the first to be in trouble. It's important to take care of our body before it gives up. Decrease the foods that enable the strong organ and increase the foods that strengthen the weaker ones.

Is it my job to understand all this?

Yes, to live this body to its fullest potential and to make upgrades to it is our responsibility. This is a personal journey into our very Self. Through observation, research, application, and practice, we seek to gain clarity on the interconnecting pieces of our physical, mental, emotional, and spiritual selves. It will tell us who we are and where we are going.

We must also be aware of how every day and every season brings external changes that affect us all, regardless of how balanced our body system is.

And while some things in us change and move with the seasons, there are things that remain unchanged and unaffected. With this observation and understanding, we can apply what we have learned to benefit and strengthen our physical, emotional, and spiritual health. It's much simpler once we understand what this is and apply it.

However, some organ body structures are very complicated and therefore difficult to identify and remedy underlying issues. It constantly changes, becoming one thing, then another. The combination of internal and external energies creates a chemical change in the body, causing the constant shifting of energies. Because it is very difficult to diagnose these body types, an expert of experts is required. Seek an expert of experts to properly understand and diagnose the existing problems, otherwise it will take a long time to fully understand and treat the underlying issues. Admittedly, there aren't many experts of this level out there.

First, have a good virtue account ready (*see* "Virtue Account," Chapter 9) to find this level of expert who is willing to help. We may be asking ourselves what a virtue account has to do with our issues. Our virtue account will create room and expand our capacity to understand, to make changes, and to grow. Without the virtue account, the expert of experts will be unable to help as we continue to spin without a landing in sight.

How Virtue Account Saves Us

Long ago, a very good friend of mine and his wife came for a visit. This man was kind-hearted, very fair, and principled. With a somber expression, he told me that after months of extensive testing, he had been diagnosed with cancer, for which there was no known cure at the time. The doctors gave him about six months to live, at best. However, he didn't want to leave his cherished wife.

"Is there any way to live longer with this cancer?" he asked.

I answered, "No. With the cancer, you won't be able to live beyond what the doctors have told you. However, if you are willing to make some adjustments to your eating habits, especially your heavy nightly snacks, you may be able to change the direction of your cancer. I will guide you through 30 days, after which you should get tested again. It should prove to you that the cancer has changed direction. However, if you think that it's all finished and you return to your old eating habits, know that the cancer will come back. If you choose to return to your cancerous life with your old eating habits, I won't be there to help you again. In other words, you must continue with your new lifestyle and eating habits if you want to live and enjoy life without cancer."

"Is that it? That's all I have to do to keep on living?" he asked, surprised.

"Yep." I replied.

I helped him, not because he was a good friend of mine, but because he had a great virtue account. My friend once had a Hispanic delivery man working part-time for him. The delivery man was eking out a living, living from day to day. One day, he became ill and had to be taken to the emergency room by my friend. There they found out that the man had cancer in its last stage. Due to the severity of his illness, the delivery man couldn't be discharged from the hospital and had to be admitted. He was given constant morphine injections to manage the terrible physical pain he was suffering. Instead of leaving the poor man to his fate, my friend made a point of visiting him for two to twelve hours every day. He sat next to the bed of the dying man, comforting and patiently listening to his life's story that was mostly filled with pain and agony, with few brief moments of brightness. He continued to listen and act as companion and witness until the man finally passed away. My friend was the only one who cared enough to attend the man's funeral. This act of kindness and compassion was an admirable deed. It was for this that I had decided to help him.

After 30 days of following my instructions, he got retested. There was no cancer to be found. The doctors told him that they must have misdiagnosed him, and encouraged him to continue whatever he was doing. My friend lived for many years with his lovely wife and eventually died of old age.

I drove three days to attend his funeral service to honor his departure. I mention this because I don't go to funerals. I don't even plan on going to my own funeral. However, I went to this one because I respected this man, and wanted to make sure that I did all I could for him and his family.

He was the most kind-hearted and principled friend I knew. He did good deeds without expecting anything in return. And yet, he did receive a return on his good deed. Because he wasn't expecting any, it came as a blessing in disguise for him. And if he didn't use the blessings of his good deed, it would be used by his close family members. The good deed would remain until it was used up completely by him or his family. The best thing about a virtue account was that, unlike money or material possessions, no one could take it away from him. It was something that only he and his family could use, with no stealing possible by anyone.

And had he done this good deed with any strings attached, it would never have counted towards his virtue account, no matter how big or well done the deed. Thankfully, my friend did all his good deeds without any conditions attached.

I once asked him what it was that made him live such a way, with honor to himself. He said, "That's the way my family lived and taught me to live. And, it is also the right thing to do as a human being."

Virtue account is thief-proof. No safe or storage is needed, with no middleman, no management fees, no account numbers, or logins. The universe remembers, unconditionally activating the Virtue Account and sending someone to assist when the need arises. Best of all, as it has no expiration date, the virtue account remains good until it's fully used. The universe always provides dividends on what's in the virtue account. It's a secure investment for ourselves and always guarantees return.

Some of us connect more strongly with logic than inner connection. But with some virtue account, someone moves to save us.

We save ourselves by listening to our own inner guidance, the gut feeling or the quiet voice within, that sometimes warns us not to proceed with something. However, some of us only listen through our logic. Luckily, someone or something intervenes to demand our attention. The following story is of such a person.

There was a man who was about to leave for an important appointment. As he was about to leave his house, he received a phone call that required his attention. He told the caller that since he was about to leave for an appointment and the matter wasn't urgent, he would deal with it after he got back.

However, the caller was adamant that he take care of the issue immediately, before anything else. The man reluctantly agreed and unhappily did the required task that he could have easily done after he returned from his appointment. The task took only ten minutes, but each minute felt like hours to him.

With the task done, the man hurried to his appointment in his car. His frustration grew when he found himself in a mile-long traffic jam. He was already late as it was. His logic began to blame the caller for the situation he was in, as this was a very important meeting for him. However, with no cell phone to inform the person he was to meet of his late arrival, he had to get there as soon as possible.

Ahead of him, there was a terrible multiple-car accident that had instantly taken five lives, with many more injured and hospitalized. When he found out, it shocked him. Without the caller, the earlier timing would have had him right in the middle of this terrible accident. All of his logical complaints against the caller suddenly ceased, and he turned inward. The man thanked the caller for saving his life.

For some of us, it takes a drastic event to get in touch with ourselves. And without a virtue account in place, he would not have taken the call, or followed through with the caller's demand.

How Can I Understand the
Signs Coming From My Body?

The body has a signal system. The first signal the body sends out is light and soft, and the second is mid-range. If there is no response to the first two signals, the third signal takes it up a notch and sends a distress signal, asking to be noticed. However, once we receive the message and understand it, the signal stops and the body releases its accumulated stress through a sigh of relief. Sending out continual messages is tremendously stressful on the body.

If no response is received, the body will try sending the signal several more times, and possibly multiple signals, before fading out like a dying battery. At this point the body has no choice but to break down since it is unable to maintain itself on its own.

At this point, the owner of the body suddenly wants to know what is going on and why, after having ignored all the SOS signals from the body. It is the responsibility of the owner to understand what has happened to their body, and if they are unable to do so, they need to take themselves to a professional to help them understand.

True, recognizing our body's signals isn't easy. This is because we are trying to understand through the logic functions of our organ system. The majority of us are absolutely clueless when it comes to our own body system. However, there are some who are conscientiously aware of all that is happening in their bodies. By being conscientiously aware, we learn to remedy the problem or search to understand the signal's meaning. And surprisingly, we often have the answers already within us.

This is same as having a car that we regularly maintain to ensure reliability and to extend the life of the car. We don't expect the individual car parts to do regular maintenance on themselves or to understand the whole car system. By maintaining the car ourselves, some of us travel long distances knowing that the car will carry us safely to our destination. While some do regular maintenance at home, most of us take the car to the experts who do this regularly for a fee. We can save lot of hassle and money if we maintain the car ourselves.

Let's take my car for example. I regularly maintain my car and do repairs as needed. It has run 240,000 miles so far, and is still going strong. I could have purchased two cars, had I not taken good care of it. Good care saved me from unnecessary car payments and hassle.

It is the same way with my body. I do regular maintenance, and if by chance

I am unable to remedy the issue, I take my body to an appropriate and experienced specialist, doctor, or practitioner who has been trained and educated in their particular field.

When my body is really sick, I don't try to dream it away. I know from past experience that ignoring the warning signals is to pay too high a price. So I try to take note of the signals as early as possible and save myself unnecessary stress and agony.

Some deluded thinkers among us believe that a car can run forever without regular maintenance or that it's someone else's job to maintain it, just like with their body. Without maintenance, a car is continuously low on gas/oil/water, which ends up burning or melting its internal parts, ruining them beyond repair.

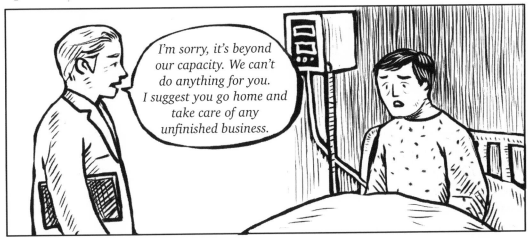

The above is a sad scenario, but this person is fortunate that he gets the chance to say goodbye to his loved ones and tidy up loose ends. We all need time to prepare for the end so we can leave with proper closure.

So, returning to the body signals, it all depends on the organs and the severity of their condition.

- If we have strong Kidneys, the female reproductive area and the heart can become affected. Our body signals to the stomach to take care of it. If we do not respond, it moves on to the breast and the female reproductive area to send out the signal. The common signal is that of always feeling cold or damp.

- If we have a strong Heart, the sequence of health problems will likely begin with Kidney/gallbladder, and then Lung/colon, followed by Stomach/spleen (depending on the condition of the supporting organs). The signals from the Kidney/gallbladder area can be tightness, headache, or pains. If these signals asking for help are ignored, the Heart system will begin to draw energy from the Lungs, colon, and bone marrow, essentially "melting" them down to survive. And if there is still no help available, the Heart will go to the Stomach.

- If we have a strong Liver, the sequence of health problems will likely begin with the Lungs, then go to Stomach/spleen. The signal often comes as a mild tightness in the chest at first, later becoming more frequent and noticeable. After many tries without any response, the Liver will go to the Stomach for more signals. There will be lot of useless mental chatter and thoughts, indicating malfunctioning of Stomach and spleen. After this, the Liver will move to another area but most of the time, it will be dealt with at the Stomach and spleen. This is a minor problem.

- If we have strong Lungs, the sequence will likely begin with the Stomach, then Liver, and then the Heart. Unless we have a Stomach that is somewhat strong, the stress on it will be very high as the walls of the Stomach begins to thin.

- If we have a very strong Stomach, the sequence of health problems will likely begin with the Kidneys, then the Liver, and then the Lungs.

If the other organs are too weak to contribute to the running of the body system, the person can die quickly from the first stage.

If the other organs are able to contribute, some people will go through a few more stages before giving up.

If the strong organ can give up some of its power to the other organs in order to support its existence during its illness, the person has a better chance of surviving, if it's not too late.

Instead of waiting for our organs to fail and send desperate signals, it is much better to prepare in advance and make the necessary adjustments to our weak and strong organs. Most of us aren't equipped or educated to deal with these kind of health emergencies. And sometimes, our thoughts and actions are dictated by our dominant organ, which makes correctly dealing with our health issues even more difficult. It is important to note that learned habits can imitate or mask the real signals sent by the body. We must use our knowledge wisely.

Is it possible that my system is unable to have the messages delivered to me?

If our organ systems are imbalanced, unable to connect, or unable to interpret the message correctly from each organ to us, we can't hear it because of faulty connections.

However, as the owner of our body, it is our duty and responsibility to make sure all the organs are equipped to communicate correctly by nurturing its needs and making adjustments on the weak and strong organs.

Our body is affected by the changes that occur every second, minute, hour, day, week, month, year, decade, 60 years, century, and so on. We may have to learn to observe the changes that happen in the days, months, and years and see if we can know the difference. We have already experienced the changes and know that they have occurred, though we may not consciously or precisely be aware of it.

To be more in tune with ourselves and build better inner connection, it's helpful to practice some meditation, yoga and Zen.

Retreat Center
for Cancer Patients

The retreat was in Yeo-Su, South Korea. It had been established decades earlier for the purpose of teaching preventative healthcare and healthy living habits, such as eating wholesome foods, doing exercise, right thinking, right prayers, honoring the body as a gift from God and using the Bible as the source of God's teaching. It was run by the SDA.

The preventative healthcare didn't take off as they had hoped. Not many people in the general public were interested in learning about preventative care or healthy living. They were busy with other things and didn't think to take care of their bodies as they should.

Instead, what the retreat center had now was a massive number of cancer patients who had come to the retreat as their last resort. This retreat was their last hope and last recourse before they expected to die.

Curiously, many found the retreat to be a healing journey for the body as well as the mind. The word got around quickly.

I called them and asked if I could enter the retreat and follow all their programs. I told them that I wanted to observe and learn in order to help people with incurable illnesses. I explained that I was in the process of understanding the root causes of cancer. Whatever they were doing to make stage-4 cancer patients well was an important missing piece that I needed in order to understand human illness.

Without knowing and understanding this piece, there was no way I could effectively help people. Working blindly was not an option. I would take only a week, I offered, while paying for the full 21-day retreat. The representative told me that they only accepted cancer patients who had medical records documenting their condition. She was firm. I had one card left to persuade the representative to let me in.

I had gone to a special school for healthcare professionals in Bakersfield, CA. It was sponsored by five generous doctors and their families who funded a trust account that provided an important education for present and future generations. They believed that their wealth wasn't theirs to begin with but belonged to God and was to be used for God's work. They believed, lived, preached, and shared their resources according to God's teachings.

The education was mainly for SDA members who were doctors, nurses, health professionals, and pastors. I wasn't any of those, but they accepted me, nevertheless.

The education provided was a heart-opening experience for me. During the four-month program, not only did they educate us; they also gave us housing, provided healthy food, clothing, and spending money. Their beliefs were based on the Bible as God's teaching, and they actually lived out what they believed.

To actually witness these people practicing what they preached was shocking. I had heard of such individuals but I had no personal experience with them. It touched my heart profoundly. I spent many nights crying silently as I walked alone, waking myself up to their deep generosity and kindness, and feeling ashamed that I had not bothered to meet them earlier. My hardened heart softened immeasurably and my eyes were opened.

I had wanted to get into the retreat to learn more, without having to mention my education at Bakersfield. But the representative wasn't going to budge, so I told her about the education, and she transferred my call to one of the resident doctors. After a few exchanges, the doctor praised the program in California and hoped that my retreat visit would help me in my search for answers and, in the future, allow me to help others in need. This was going to be his contribution to my journey.

In 2001, I entered the retreat center where cancer patients were allowed to stay for only 21 days. There were no extensions nor exceptions to the rules. However, early checkout was possible.

It was located in an ideal place to have a retreat. The place felt secure, calm, and peaceful. The buildings of the retreat center faced the bay, with low mountains rising on either side like two protective arms. By feng shui standards, one couldn't ask for a better setting for a retreat center.

This beautiful place was filled with mostly cancer patients who had run out of all other options. This center was their last hope. I had never seen so many cancer patients in one place. Everyone was critically ill with various types of cancer.

Some could barely walk, and others had to be supported to move around. I alone looked healthy among all the other participants entering that day.

Four people were assigned to each room, without exception. The retreat was in high demand with a long waiting list that could stretch for months. No matter who they were, or how wealthy or powerful, everyone shared rooms.

Most of the workers there were volunteers. Some were there to simply serve the sick while others were there to learn how to take care of their sick family members back home.

On quiet nights, I heard the many anguished cries of pain and suffering. There were also a lot of prayers.

One voice pleaded, "God, please take me now. I can't take this pain anymore."

Another sobbed, "Why are you punishing me...?"

This one desperately beseeched, "I'm sorry for all the wrongs I have done. I will not do them anymore. I promise. Just take my pain away...please! Please!"

This went on for a while, each speaking directly to their God or Judge, pleading their case. Some of them continued to blame, curse, and cry all night. What nights they were!

I noticed that some people were looking better with each passing day. And then there were those few who decided to leave on the second day, disappointed that they didn't heal instantly like they saw on television.

The place was clean and modern, staffed with warm, kind and professional people who worked to help any way they could. The food was buffet style, where you served yourself. It was wholesome, with homegrown organic vegetables and no processed food in sight. Some people complained of having paid a lot of money for this retreat and getting only rabbit food to eat. They just wanted to eat their regular foods that had made them sick in the first place.

Every morning we gathered in the courtyard to do stretches, waking up all the parts of our body. After the meals, we had to walk to the mountain behind the center, each carrying a bottle of water. Some couldn't walk more than ten steps at a time. The helper assisting the person would wait for him/her to recover before resuming the walk. The cancer patients continued to look better each day.

During one of my sunbathing times on the secured rooftop patio with a fantastic view of the bay, I encountered a woman who was in the last stage of liver cancer. She was there by herself, soaking up the sun. Not many chose to sunbathe at the retreat.

I was trying to distance myself and give us both some privacy when she waved and invited me closer.

"You're not going to scream, are you?" I asked her.

With a warm smile she replied, "I'm not contagious by any means, and no, I will not scream or bite."

She said she sunbathed every morning and that this was part of her treatment. She found the whole sunbathing experience very soothing for some reason. Lying completely naked, she made sure to rotate her body like a rotisserie chicken so the sun could penetrate every inch of her body as much as possible.

Her story was that this was her second stint at the retreat center and she almost didn't get invited back. The first time she arrived, she was at death's door. Her family had brought her here, grasping at even the remotest chance to save her. Though she wasn't a religious person, her parents were.

She recovered quickly during the 21 days of retreat. When her family came to pick her up at the end of the retreat, they had come bracing themselves for the worst outcome. They had prayed for her healing everyday, but if God chose otherwise, they would have to accept. So when they saw her looking healthy, they were amazed.

The first 21 days of retreat had provided great results. Because she had improved, she followed what she learned from the retreat with all her family supporting her. Sometime later, her doctor declared her cancer-free. At last, she had beat the cancer.

She was so happy and excited that she immediately returned to her pre-cancer lifestyle—the very lifestyle that had led her to cancer in the first place. She forgot all about healthy living.

Soon, she began to notice that her body system wasn't working right and her health beginning to deteriorate. By the time she went to see her doctor, she received news that her cancer was back with a vengeance and she didn't have much time left on her body's clock.

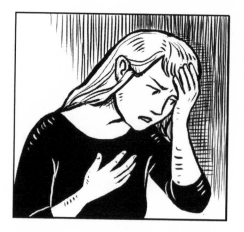

The news hit her hard. Once cured, then shouldn't she have stayed cured?

This would be true if she had stayed free and clear of the toxic and damaging lifestyle she had inflicted on her mind and body. She had not realized this and had brought herself back to the same dire predicament as before. She had to wake up from this bad dream. Realizing her mistake, she wanted to get well again.

She called the retreat center, but they were reluctant to accept her. There was no space available, they said. She pondered for a day before deciding to drive to the center regardless of space availability. She had no time to lose and she hoped that a spot would open up for her. She had to get well and this time she was determined to stick with healthy living. All the things they taught her, she would follow conscientiously for the long haul.

When she arrived at the center, she was told that someone had just vacated a spot. Without thinking, she blurted out, "Thank God, I am saved!"

And that was two weeks ago, she said. Before she had left home, she had told her friends to consider her dead. This was because she had to live and get well. She wasn't going to mess up this time with her old lifestyle. She was going to attentively follow the program and learn to enjoy every moment of it.

Failure was not an option this time, and once and for all she was going to be responsible for herself. She began to allow herself to understand and completely surrender to it. She felt deep peace.

She felt the changes in her body system, which came to life a little more each day. This time she was grateful for everything. The first time, she had come because she was dying and there hadn't been much of a choice. Her family had brought her here out of desperate hope.

Now, she thanked God for the second chance, though she still wasn't religious. She said, "I was lucky this time. I was *very* lucky, this time." She quietly repeated this several times to herself. There was calm and peace in her demeanor.

She was very fortunate to wake up from her old habits. This experience was what it took to shake her awake and for her to finally live life with deep appreciation, gratitude, and dignity. She was lucky, indeed, because most of us don't wake up even with this kind of wake-up call.

Now, through realizations, determination, self-love, and self-respect, her old habits only come for an occasional visit. She is now under the wake-up master at work. The functions and habits of her dominant organs can't demand their old way of living anymore. She knows all too well where that road leads. So when the old thoughts arise, she only acknowledges and smiles at the old habits, and does not follow.

It would have been better if she had first loved herself.
It would have been better if she had taken preventative measures earlier on. And it would have been better if she had not waited until the last moment to get well.

But it could have been her inner programming or her stubbornness that had prevented her from loving herself before. Still, it is far better that she came back to life with a profound realization and now finally knows to love herself and receive love in return.

Experience every day as a blessed day to make upgrades to ourselves.

Know and accept that everyone can connect to their higher self.

Everything comes and goes, and can peacefully flow with the passing seasons.

Every day, fully focus on committing to the present moment.

Chapter 2

The Nature of Organs

The Nature of Organs and Their Functions

Our organ system follows the physical laws of nature.

The organs are part of us, and they play an intricate part in who we are and what we accomplish. Importantly, our organs also serve to take us where we need to go. So it's crucial that we understand and take care of our organ system. If one of the organs becomes sick, the rest will suffer as well. Sometimes other organs are able to provide the support and get by, but sometimes the sick organ is the only one capable of providing what we need. Without the support of all the organs, we will be functionally crippled, unable to receive, perceive, and decode the messages that come to us internally and externally.

When one of the organs become sick, it may be easily fixed or may take a while depending on the individual. However, for the most part it is fixable.

As we come to understand our body system, we will know which part of that system is in trouble, what part of the organ is off, and how to solve it. Otherwise, we will continue to struggle with the disharmony of our body system and go nowhere in our life's journey.

Understand how each organ connects to different parts of our body and know each organ's function. The following are the ten organs and their functions.

The Five Organs

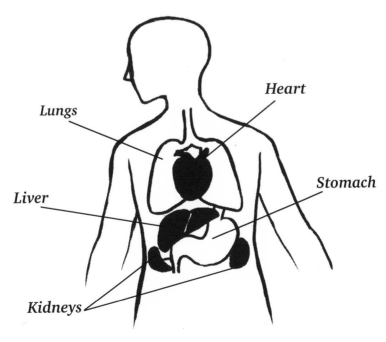

The Connecting Organs

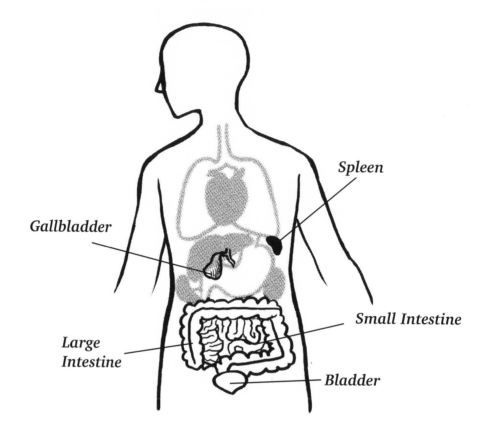

Spleen

Gallbladder

Large Intestine

Small Intestine

Bladder

The Main Five Organs + Connecting Organs

Kidney and Bladder = ear/sound = bone marrow

Heart and Small Intestine = tongue/taste = nerves/blood vessels

Liver and Gallbladder = eyes/sight = tendons/muscles

Lung and Large Intestine = nose/smell = skin

Stomach and Spleen = mouth/thought = thigh/knee

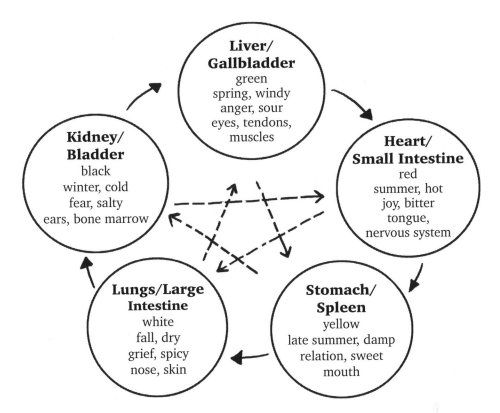

The sixth organ is not listed here. It is invisible but functions like the visible organs. The sixth organ is crucial to our existence here and now, and beyond.

Kidney/Water

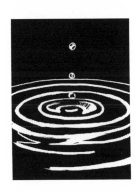

Color: Black
Direction: North

It is dark, hidden from the light.

Helps and regulates growth, and provides energies to all organs. It holds the life energy. The Kidney supports bones, bone marrow, hearing, hormones, and reproductive organs and genitals.

The Kidney energy pushes away with "+" and "–". Its tendency is to spread outward, just as water flows over the land and soaks the earth.

Its season is winter and it is damp, preparing for the coming of spring. It is this energy that allows the spring life to grow.

This energy also holds, representing life and death, and softening of things. It is full of knowledge, making for a scientific mind that researches and improves, bringing positive ideas to the table. It has a way of smoothing things out in a softening way. And because it is damp, it can create mold in the systems if not properly circulated.

Heart/Fire

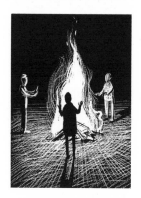

Color: Red
Direction: South

All energy goes outward. Inside is empty.

The Heart governs the circulatory system and the nervous system.

The Heart energy sparks when "+" and "−" meet. It is attractive and because people love beautiful and gorgeous things, people fall madly in love with it.

The season is summer, and like the sun/fire, it brightens the space around them. But also like fire, it desires to consume and burn everything around it, including the person who has it.

Fire energy looks fantastic on the outside, but inside there's a struggle. It is very greedy, and it only goes up. Talented in an artistic way, fire nature appears passionate, energetic, and intuitive. It can also be explosive and over-heated, destroying the cooling system. However, if the cooling system works properly, it will have a different outcome.

Liver/Wood

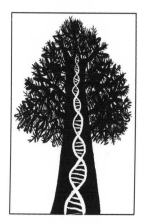

Color: Blue/Green
Direction: East

It sprouts and calmly grows tall in agile, upward movement.

It holds blood and manages moisture metabolism, eyes, muscles, tendons, joints, fingernails and toenails.

When Liver energy has "+" and "−" in harmony, it becomes competitive and seeks improvement and growth. The wood nature likes prestige and is soft, kind, and warm when it is harmonized.

The Liver energy is generally tall, slender, and gentle. It symbolizes spring when everything comes to life. The spring weather is nice, warm, soft, and gentle.

Liver and gallbladder is like a sprout of new growth. When a part is used, it will grow back, constantly replenishing itself. This person's Liver system will continue to heal.

Lung/Metal

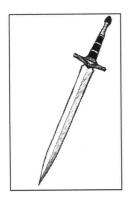

Color: White
Direction: West

Cool, fair, disciplined, time of ripening and harvest

The Lungs control the breath, the original energy, and all energies from food. It also governs the skin, nose, respiratory system, and the motor nervous system. It is weak against cold and heat.

The Lung energy pulls with "+" and "–", a strong contracting force. It is hard, forceful, and powerful.

Its season is fall, therefore it represents harvesting.

When combined with the Heart/fire energy, it exercises fair judgement. With the strength and softness coexisting, it knows *what* to do and *what not* to do. It understands the dark side of human nature as well as its weaknesses, coming to people's aid when needed. Principle is more important than money for this energy and can make other people nervous.

Stomach/Earth

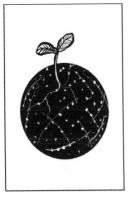

Color: Yellow
Direction: Center/ Southwest

It is the center that gathers, where all things are transformed and allowed to grow.

The Stomach produces and absorbs all the nutrients the body needs, and gives rise to the source that creates life.

This energy connects "+" and "–", and in doing so, creates harmony and unity. It has a tendency to hold and embrace all things.

The Stomach sits at the center, and the four seasons circle around it, making all things grow. Through its changes come the finished product. We plant, grow, and then harvest. This is what the earth-energy person provides, with the help of four other elements. It makes the body a bit dull because the earth energy draws everything in, embracing it all in a chaotic way.

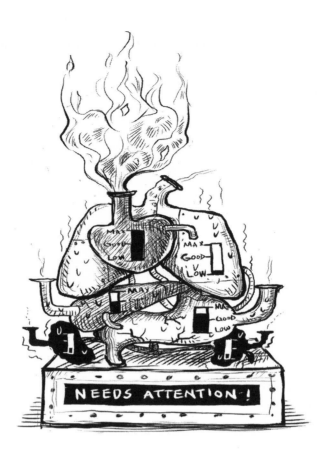

We are much more than our organ systems. However, most illnesses stem from the five disharmonized energy systems.

By working on the underlying organ issues, most of these illnesses can be treated.

So it's important that we know which part of our body is off and know how to resolve it. Otherwise, we will simply struggle with the disharmony and go nowhere.

The following provides some examples of organ function and its symptoms.

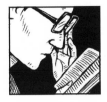

Someone who wears glasses often has weak Liver or excess Lung energy.

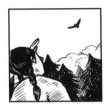

Someone with good vision likely has a healthy Liver system.

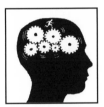

Someone who thinks too much likely has weak Stomach/spleen.

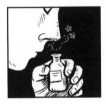

Someone with a very keen sense of smell likely has strong Lung energy.

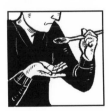

Someone who can't taste likely has Heart-related problems.

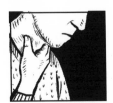

Someone with ear/throat issues likely has weak Kidney energy.

The Five Organs and Their Manifestations

The unique combination of energies in a person ultimately decides the outcome. The following describes the energies individually and the way they manifest in a person.

Kidney

A person with strong Kidneys has excess water energy. The body is built to have continuous water energy coming into it. Because their bodies are invaded by excess water energy, this person will likely invade other people's spaces — be they physical or mental. Like water, they will find a way to flow through and around obstacles, driven by blind desire to keep going.

This also happens in the body. The excess water energy flows into other organs, interfering with the functions of the Stomach, Lung, Heart, and possibly Liver. This disrupts the regular functioning of the body systems. This particular energy causes people to be talkative, invasive, fearful, disrespectful, mistrusting, and full of doubt.

With this kind of body, the person will often have stomach problems, and if female, will have problems with the reproductive system. Too much excess Kidney energy will put out the Heart/fire, overrunning it, and potentially causing the individual to die in their sleep.

The way to improve this condition is to eat sweet and bitter foods. Although the water energy seeks foods with cold elements to them, one must avoid them all. The more one consumes it, the sicker the body will become.

Heart

When someone has excess Heart energy, they tend to be attractive, love to go shopping, and desire to keep going up, and up, and up. They cannot come down and get easily depressed.

With excess heart energy, their Kidney system is weak. They look prettier on the outside. Inside, they deal with negativity, depression, and reproductive organ problems. This type of person requires an audience to live on. And without that audience, they often collapse and fall into depression.

This particular energy pattern will also explode, due to an engine that runs too hot and the lack of "cooling system" (think Kidneys). This body structure only wants to live in a shiny, high-profile public lifestyle.

If they want to maintain that kind of life and live longer, they must maintain their cooling system. This is essential. They must do this by avoiding all sweet and bitter foods.

Liver

A person with excess Liver system is genuinely kind, but is irresponsible and indecisive. It takes a long time for them to make a decision, and they are not always clear.

Excessive Liver energy will weaken the Stomach. Unable to bring themselves back up, they will often face depression-like symptoms if they lack Lung energy.

For a person with this body structure to have credibility and decisiveness, they must strengthen their Lung power. This person is very intellectual, does lots of research, and reads a lot of books. They tend to be stubborn and, typically, a know-it-all. When they strengthen their Lung and Heart energies, they become very noble.

They can improve their situation by eating beef, fish, lamb, and spicy foods. However, other proteins must be avoided despite their intellect telling them otherwise. It doesn't know the body's excesses.

Lung

Someone with good Lung power is principled, precise, and opinionated. Though they are not warm and sweet, they do the morally correct thing. And because they do the right thing, they believe kindness is not necessary. They have a heroic mindset and are benefited greatly by Heart/fire energy.

Excess Lung weakens the Liver, causing the Stomach, Liver, and Heart to work continuously. This creates stress on the whole system, which in turn causes the person to become impatient. Though the Lung, untempered by the other organs, is able to see and take action, things don't happen as intended.

In most cases, this particular person does not have empathy or sympathy for others. We find this type often serving as CEOs or military officers. If this person strengthens their Heart and Liver energy, they become like a finely honed sword. However, without these energies, they become blunt and rough around the edges, with people afraid to be near them.

Though this energy type loves beef, fish, and anything spicy, they must avoid eating them in order to improve their situation.

Stomach

A person with excess Stomach energy is a collector. They collect anything and everything at all cost, throwing away nothing. They love money and collect anything related to money in order to gain more. This body's organ structure also craves "free things."

Excess Stomach energy causes acidity and Kidney problems where the Kidney does not function properly. The circulation slows down, and the body tries to hold everything in as much as possible.

To improve, they need to eat bitter foods and foods that have cold and clear elemental properties. And by providing their body with a regular supply of Kidney energy, they can attain the wealth they so desire.

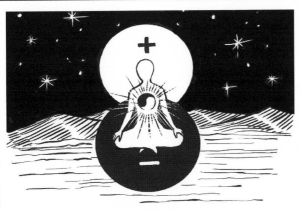

We have heaven, earth, and all living things, including humans.

The heaven's energy and the earth's energy circulate and flow through us, connecting the "+" (positive charge) and the "−" (negative charge) through our body. When connected correctly, it sparks, flows, and harmonizes.

According to ancient legends, heaven is "+" and earth is "−". Together they control all things and create change. The "+" and the "−" carry divine energy that gives life and nurtures that life. Therefore, when our human bodies and all living things harmonize through the yin-yang, most illnesses can be fixed.

These are examples of yin and yang.

Yin	Moon	Woman	Earth
Yang	Sun	Man	Heaven

Kidney
Urinary/Bladder
WATER
Salty

Liver
Gallbladder
WOOD
Sour

Heart
Small Intestine
FIRE
Bitter

Lung
Large Intestine
METAL
Spicy

Stomach
Spleen
EARTH
Sweet

The Nature of the Universe

Within all of us exist all sentient beings. Not only do we carry traits based on our DNA, but also all other traits that we consider good, bad, ugly, cunning, manipulative, etc. Only when we are awakened to all these things, do they dissolve.

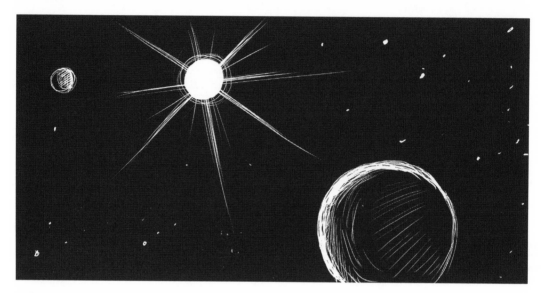

Where does this Nature of Organs and Function theory come from?

This particular theory appeared in ancient Gojoseon. Hermits living deep in the forest developed ancient medicine and with awakening eyes saw the movements of the stars and the changing seasons. They saw how they were connected, and thus established the Chun-moon (astrological) theory.

What the Chun-moon theory describes existed from the beginning of time. People simply realized this and it was put into writing.

They saw beneath the surface and began to read the land, mountains, rivers, and seas, and thus established the Ji-ri (feng shui) geomantic theory.

These people also read the human body structure. They saw in it a small universe where all the organs and meridians were interconnected, each playing a role in how it functioned together.

This is what we now know as Eastern medicine.

Chapter 3

Organs and Their Symptoms

Strong Kidneys

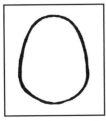

Each body organ exhibits characteristics unique to itself. This individual with strong Kidney organs has major attachments/traits as follows:

Intelligent/Flows like water

You may have noticed these symptoms in yourself or in others. The list of symptoms for someone with strong Kidney energy is as follows:

Physical Symptoms:

- lack of energy
- hot flashes
- Stomach issues
- breast issues
- reproductive issues
- sluggishness
- tiredness
- weak Heart/small intestine (biggest)
- withdrawn at times
- feels cold most of the time

Behavioral Symptoms:

- very talkative, tries to dominate most situations
- sharply opinionated
- rude/unkind
- prone to negativity
- anxiety
- selfish/inconsiderate
- thinks too much
- above normal appetite for sex
- loves sweets
- strong research skills
- often works in the IT, research and science fields, and service industries
- shy/timid

If these warning symptoms are ignored, depending on the condition of other organs, it will lead to Kidney, Stomach, Heart and Liver problems.

What will help ease the problem?

See "How to Improve My Health," Chapter 6

What's the benefit?

- more energy and confidence
- greater clarity
- a calm body
- is more considerate
- look younger
- regular and happy bowel movements
- better sleep

Strong Kidney-Kidney

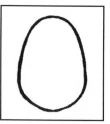

Each body organ exhibits characteristics unique to itself. This individual with very strong Kidney organs has major attachments/ traits as follows:

Sexy/Overconfident/Overflowing

You may have noticed these symptoms in yourself or in others. The list of symptoms for someone with very strong Kidney energy is as follows:

Physical Symptoms:

- lack of energy
- hot flashes
- Stomach issues
- breast issues
- reproductive issues
- often feels cold

- blood clot
- tiredness
- weak Heart/small intestine (biggest)
- withdrawn at times
- submerged in water energy
- circulation issues

Behavioral Symptoms:

- very talkative, tries to dominate most conversations
- sharply opinionated
- rude/unkind
- flows
- anxious/nervous/agitated
- thinks too much (brain spins excessively)

- selfish/inconsiderate
- no compassion for others
- sharp cutting thoughts
- prone to negativity
- weak center
- strong fears
- stubborn
- afraid of water

If these warning symptoms are ignored, depending on the condition of other organs, it will lead to Kidney, Heart, Stomach and Liver problems.

What will help ease the problem?

See** "How to Improve My Health," Chapter 6

What's the benefit?

- more energy and confidence
- greater clarity
- a calmer body

- look younger
- better sleep
- more considerate
- more stable

Strong Kidney-Heart

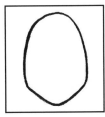

Each body organ exhibits characteristics unique to itself. This individual with strong Kidney-Heart organs has major attachments/traits as follows:

Extremely bright/Popular as a public figure

You may have noticed these symptoms in yourself or in others. The list of symptoms for someone with strong Kidney-Heart energy is as follows:

Physical Symptoms:

- weak Lungs/large intestine (biggest)
- lack of energy
- hot flashes
- lack of mental sharpness
- tiredness
- withdrawn at times

Behavioral Symptoms:

- prone to suicidal thoughts
- nervous/anxious
- appears bright on the outside
- romantic (attractive)
- lacks drive, decisiveness
- sadness/depression inside
- sociable
- popular
- weak sense of reality

If these warning symptoms are ignored, depending on the condition of other organs, it will lead to Lung, Liver, and Stomach problems.

*When this individual has suicidal thoughts, it indicates the depletion of his/her Lung energy. The Lung is basically dying out, unable to provide staying power to support the body system.

What will help ease the problem?

See "How to Improve My Health," Chapter 6

What's the benefit?

- more energy and confidence
- greater clarity
- calmer body
- more centered
- regular and happy bowel movements
- better sleep
- returns to reality

Strong Kidney-Liver

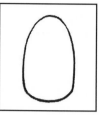 Each body organ exhibits characteristics unique to itself. This individual with strong Kidney-Liver organs has major attachments/traits as follows:

Persistence/Integrity/Superb intelligence

You may have noticed these symptoms in yourself or in others. The list of symptoms for someone with strong Kidney-Liver energy is as follows:

Physical Symptoms:

- lack of energy
- Lung problems
- lack of mental sharpness
- digestive problems
- Heart issues
- body tends to run cold
- Stomach/spleen issues (biggest)
- tiredness
- withdrawn at times due to weak Lung support
- balance problems
- weak nervous system

Behavioral Symptoms:

- tendency towards negative thoughts
- very talkative
- a bit timid/shy
- very witty
- are often genius professionals
- humane
- very intelligent
- good business sense, planning/design
- lacks flexibility/adaptability
- a strong head for finances
- likes cleanliness
- anxiety
- thinks excessively
- nervous, agitated

If these warning symptoms are ignored, depending on the condition of other organs, it will lead to Lung and Kidney problems.

What will help ease the problem?

See "How to Improve My Health," Chapter 6

What's the benefit?

- more energy
- sharpness of mind
- a calm body
- fewer worries
- expansion of view
- stability

Strong Kidney-Lung

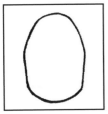

Each body organ exhibits characteristics unique to itself. This individual with strong Kidney-Lung organs has major attachments/traits as follows:

Principled/Independent/Extremely intelligent thinker (genius-like)

You may have noticed these symptoms in yourself or in others. The list of symptoms for someone with strong Kidney-Lung energy is as follows:

Physical Symptoms:

- sensitive colon
- Heart/small intestine issues (biggest)
- Stomach/spleen issues
- digestive problems
- back problems
- problem with circulation
- joint stiffness
- catches cold easily
- slightly feverish at times
- unable to warm up easily
- tiredness
- shortness of breath

Behavioral Symptoms:

- cold/lack of kindness
- sharp mind when it comes to money, computer, and sex
- can be cute and charming
- extravagant/vain
- very logical
- independent
- selfish
- prefers to be alone
- has very high opinion of oneself
- anxiety
- charismatic

If these warning symptoms are ignored, it will lead to continued Stomach dryness, spleen discomfort, Kidney, kidney stone, reproductive, and pancreatic problems.

What will help ease the problem?

See "How to Improve My Health," Chapter 6

What's the benefit?

- less back pain
- less cold
- a bit kinder
- more energy
- warmer
- less harsh towards oneself and others
- less stomach issues

Strong Kidney-Stomach

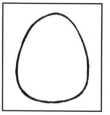

Each body organ exhibits characteristics unique to itself. This individual with strong Kidney-Stomach organs has major attachments/traits as follows:

Flows with money/Attracted to sunny people with strong Heart energy

You may have noticed these symptoms in yourself or in others. The list of symptoms for someone with strong Kidney-Stomach energy is as follows:

Physical Symptoms:

- lack of energy
- breast issues
- very weak Heart and small intestine function (biggest)
- tiredness
- withdrawn at times
- often feels cold
- circulation issues

Behavioral Symptoms:

- very talkative, tries to dominate most conversations
- unkind opinions
- rude/unkind
- often anxious and unhappy
- lack of sincere appreciation
- unable to have a bubbly personality
- anxiety
- selfish/inconsiderate
- no compassion for others
- prone to negativity
- a bit timid/shy
- very manipulative
- above normal appetite for sex and money
- extraordinary research skills
- tend to work in IT, research and science fields, and service industries
- cold and calculating

If these warning symptoms are ignored, depending on the condition of other organs, it will lead to Heart problems.

What will help ease the problem?

See "How to Improve My Health," Chapter 6

What's the benefit?

- more energy
- greater clarity
- a calm body
- is more considerate
- warm and stable
- look younger
- regular and happy bowel movements
- better sleep

Strong Heart

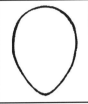

Each body organ exhibits characteristics unique to itself. This individual with strong Heart organ has major attachments/traits as follows:

Beauty/Needs to be at the center of attention/ Shopping

You may have noticed these symptoms in yourself or in others. The list of symptoms for someone with strong Heart energy is as follows:

Physical Symptoms:

- dry lips and skin
- dry Stomach
- can't digest well
- constipation
- forgets easily
- hot flashes
- depression
- body discomfort
- lack of mental sharpness
- breathing issues

- coughing
- weak Lungs/large intestine (biggest)
- slight fever (inside body)
- desire to lay down/sleep when alone
- body feels lazy but is able to go shopping
- easily tired except when at the center of attention
- thyroid issues

- feels like an inflating balloon, ready to pop
- tightness of airways, blood vessels
- shortness of breath
- tight itchy throat
- tightness of ovaries, Kidneys
- discomfort while urinating
- air bubble in urine
- nose, wrist, anus and chest issues

Behavioral Symptoms:

- sadness/depression
- prone to suicidal thoughts
- entertainer (actor/actress)

- creative
- visual
- natural artist

- weak at finishing tasks/things
- weak at managing finances
- embellishes stories/descriptions

If these warning symptoms are ignored, depending on the condition of other organs, it will lead to thyroid, breast, brain tumor, reproductive and pancreatic problems.

*When this individual has suicidal thoughts, it indicates the depletion of his/her Lung energy. The Lung is basically dying out, unable to provide staying power to support the body system.

What will help ease the problem?

See "How to Improve My Health," Chapter 6

What's the Benefit?

- body cools down
- no more foggy mind
- clarity
- calms the body
- better sleep
- balanced with radiant beauty

- softer skin (for stronger skin, taking fish products recommended)
- regular and happy bowel movements

Strong Heart-Kidney

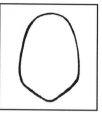

Each body organ exhibits characteristics unique to itself. This individual with strong Heart-Kidney organs has major attachments/traits as follows:

Charming/Warm/Genius inventor

You may have noticed these symptoms in yourself or in others. The list of symptoms for someone with strong Heart-Kidney energy is as follows:

Physical Symptoms:

- weak Lungs/large intestine (biggest)
- lack of energy
- hot flashes
- doesn't digest well
- lack of mental sharpness
- gets easily tired
- withdrawn at times
- a swift mind but no deep consideration

Behavioral Symptoms:

- appears bright on the outside
- prone to suicidal thoughts
- anxiety
- innovative
- intelligent
- sadness/depression in the inside
- inventor
- appears quiet, rational, warm
- spiritual

If these warning symptoms are ignored, depending on the condition of other organs, it will lead to Lung, Liver, and Stomach problems.

*When this individual has suicidal thoughts, it indicates the depletion of his/her Lung energy. The Lung is basically dying out, unable to provide staying power to support the body system.

What will help ease the problem?

See "How to Improve My Health," Chapter 6

What's the benefit?

- more energy
- greater clarity
- a calm body
- regular and happy bowel movements
- confident
- more in touch with reality
- more active
- better sleep

Strong Heart-Heart

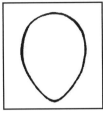 Each body organ exhibits characteristics unique to itself. This individual with very strong Heart organ has major attachments/traits as follows:

Beauty/Must be the center of attention/Shopping

You may have noticed these symptoms in yourself or in others. The list of symptoms for someone with very strong Heart energy is as follows:

Physical Symptoms:

- dry lips and skin
- dry Stomach
- hot flashes
- constipation
- indigestion
- tight itchy throat
- shortness of breath
- discomfort in the body
- weak bone/skin
- thyroid issues

- tightness of airways, blood vessels
- slightly elevated body temperature
- slight fever (inside body)
- lack of mental sharpness
- desire to lay down/sleep
- body feels lazy but is able to go shopping
- extremities feel cold

- easily tired except when at the center of attention
- feels like an inflating balloon, ready to pop
- tightness of ovaries, Kidneys
- discomfort while urinating
- air bubble in urine
- weak Lung/large intestine (biggest)

Behavioral Symptoms:

- prone to suicidal thoughts
- stubborn
- very negative (inside)
- depression

- sad/tragic
- artistic
- out of touch with reality

- public figure—a bright warm light to the masses
- movie star/entertainer

If these warning symptoms are ignored, depending on the condition of other organs, it will lead to thyroid, breast, brain tumor, reproductive and pancreatic problems.

*When this individual has suicidal thoughts, it indicates the depletion of his/her Lung energy. The Lung is basically dying out, unable to provide staying power to support the body system.

What will help ease the problem?

See "How to Improve My Health," Chapter 6

What's the benefit?

- body cools down
- no more foggy mind
- greater clarity
- calms the body
- better sleep

- softer skin
- balanced with radiant beauty
- regular and happy bowel movements
- no fire in the eyes, face, body

Strong Heart-Liver

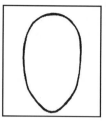

Each body organ exhibits characteristics unique to itself. This individual with strong Heart-Liver organs has major attachments/traits as follows:

Beauty/Kindness/Warmth

You may have noticed these symptoms in yourself or in others. The list of symptoms for someone with strong Heart-Liver energy is as follows:

Physical Symptoms:

- lack of energy
- hot flashes
- doesn't digest well
- lack of mental sharpness
- weak Lung/large intestine (biggest)
- constipation
- tiredness
- withdrawn at times
- rheumatism/arthritis
- weak bone/skin
- thyroid issues

Behavioral symptoms:

- often lives in fantasyland
- depression
- impractical
- soft
- gentle
- empathetic
- out of touch with reality
- very strong focus

If these warning symptoms are ignored, depending on the condition of other organs, it will lead to Lung and Kidney problems.

What will help ease the problem?

See "How to Improve My Health," Chapter 6

What's the Benefit?

- more energy
- greater clarity
- a calm body
- regular and happy bowel movements
- better sleep

Strong Heart-Lung

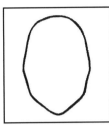

Each body organ exhibits characteristics unique to itself. This individual with strong Heart-Lung organs has major attachments/traits as follows:

Able to see beyond the obvious/An excellent investigator

You may have noticed these symptoms in yourself or in others. The list of symptoms for someone with strong Heart-Lung energy is as follows:

Physical Symptoms:

- hot flashes
- doesn't digest well
- constipation
- Liver/gall bladder problem (biggest)
- tiredness at times
- lack of energy
- muscle pain
- Kidney issues
- Stomach issues

Behavioral Symptoms:

- active
- a roller-coaster life
- absence of kindness
- impatient
- fast-moving mind
- very critical
- excited for new things
- less compassionate toward others
- able to read between the lines
- very strong focus
- intelligent

If you ignore these warning symptoms and depending on the condition of your other organs, it can lead to major health crisis due to problems with the Liver, Kidney and Stomach organs.

What will help ease the problem?

See** "How to Improve My Health," Chapter 6

How will I benefit?

- fully energized
- regular and happy bowel movements
- better sleep
- overall calmness
- wider clarity

Strong Heart-Stomach

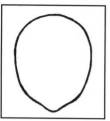

Each body organ exhibits characteristics unique to itself. This individual with strong Heart-Stomach organs has major attachments/traits as follows:

Beauty first/Greedy for spending money

You may have noticed these symptoms in yourself or in others. The list of symptoms for someone with strong Heart-Stomach energy is as follows:

Physical Symptoms:

- dry lips and skin
- dry Stomach
- can't digest well due to lack of fluids
- constipation
- forgets easily
- hot flashes
- depression
- body discomfort
- weak Kidney/bladder (biggest)

- slightly elevated body temperature
- slight fever (inside body)
- desire to lay down/sleep
- body feels lazy but is able to go shopping
- easily tired except when at the center of attention
- possible diabetes
- lack of mental sharpness
- thyroid issues

- feels like an inflating balloon, ready to pop
- tightness of airways, blood vessels
- shortness of breath
- tight itchy throat
- tightness of ovaries, Kidneys
- discomfort while urinating
- air bubble in urine
- rheumatism/arthritis

Behavioral Symptoms:

- prone to suicidal thoughts
- natural artist
- entertainer
- spender/show off
- silver tongue

- very negative
- weak at finishing tasks/things
- weak at managing finances
- beauty on the outside, hollow inside
- brings people together

If these warning symptoms are ignored, depending on the condition of other organs, it will lead to thyroid, breast, brain tumor, reproductive and pancreatic problems.

*When this individual has suicidal thoughts, it indicates the depletion of his/her Lung energy. The Lung is basically dying out, unable to provide staying power to support the body system.

What will help ease the problem?

See "How to Improve My Health," Chapter 6

What's the Benefit?

- body cools down
- clarity
- calm
- better sleep

- softer skin
- regular and happy bowel movements
- down to earth

Strong Liver

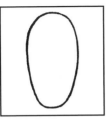

Each body organ exhibits characteristics unique to itself. This individual with strong Liver organ has major attachments/traits as follows:

Thirst for deep and vast knowledge/Prestige/ Integrity

You may have noticed these symptoms in yourself or in others. The list of symptoms for someone with strong Liver energy is as follows:

Physical Symptoms:

- Lung/large intestine/ colon problems
- feeling of sadness/ depression
- Stomach/spleen problems (biggest)
- chest discomfort
- occasionally withdrawn due to weak Lung support
- lack of mental sharpness
- weak Heart function
- tiredness
- can't digest well
- negative thoughts
- lack of energy
- possible diabetes/ arthritis

Behavioral Symptoms:

- kind
- not easily angered
- compassionate and considerate of others
- persistent but weak finish
- has difficulty entrusting work/ issues to others
- stubborn
- obsessive and paranoid
- good memory system
- excellent planner
- good at nurturing and teaching
- intelligent
- weak sense of reality
- thinks excessively

If these warning symptoms are ignored, depending on the condition of other organs, it will lead to Stomach, Lung, and Heart problems.

What will help ease the problem?

See "How to Improve My Health," Chapter 6

What's the benefit?

- more energy
- greater clarity
- open and upright chest
- more harmonious
- confident
- more independent
- better sleep

Strong Liver-Kidney

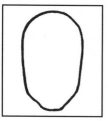

Each body organ exhibits characteristics unique to itself. This individual with strong Liver-Kidney organs has major attachments/traits as follows:

Integrity/Intelligence/Persistence

You may have noticed these symptoms in yourself or in others. The list of symptoms for someone with strong Liver-Kidney energy is as follows:

Physical Symptoms:

- Stomach/spleen problems (biggest)
- lack of energy
- Lung problems
- digestive problems
- weak Heart
- withdrawn at times due to weak Lung support
- negative thoughts
- lack of mental sharpness
- anxiety
- tiredness

Behavioral Symptoms:

- paranoid delusions
- tendency towards negative thoughts
- honest
- distrustful, but tendency to follow others easily
- thinks too much
- impractical
- intelligent
- weak finish
- stubborn
- narrow views
- calm and rational
- strong endurance
- antisocial
- conservative
- inflexible
- stuck in oneself
- decent, kind, gentle
- anxiety
- weak center/unstable

If these warning symptoms are ignored, depending on the condition of other organs, it will lead to Stomach, Heart, and Lung problems.

What will help ease the problem?

See** "How to Improve My Health," Chapter 6

What's the benefit?

- more energy
- sharpness of mind
- a calm body
- less worries
- expansion of view

Strong Liver-Heart

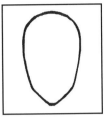

Each body organ exhibits characteristics unique to itself. This individual with strong Liver-Heart organs has major attachments/ traits as follows:

Integrity/Beauty/Compassion

You may have noticed these symptoms in yourself or in others. The list of symptoms for someone with strong Liver-Heart energy is as follows:

Physical Symptoms:

- lack of energy
- tiredness
- lack of mental sharpness
- digestive problems
- hot flashes
- thyroid issues

- bone/teeth issues
- Lung/large intestine issues (biggest)
- withdrawn at times due to weak Lung support

- occasional constipation
- respiratory issues
- rheumatism/arthritis
- diabetes

Behavioral Symptoms:

- dreamy/not grounded in reality
- hollow inside
- doesn't listen to other people's advice

- soft/kind
- negative at times
- impractical
- indecisive

- unmotivated
- rely on thoughts that pop up, not deep considerations

If these warning symptoms are ignored, depending on the condition of other organs, it will lead to Lung and Kidney problems.

What will help ease the problem?

See "How to Improve My Health," Chapter 6

What's the benefit?

- more energy
- sharpness of mind
- a calm body
- more practical

Strong Liver-Liver

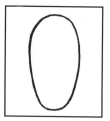

Each body organ exhibits characteristics unique to itself. This individual with very strong Liver organ has major attachments/ traits as follows:

Thirst for knowledge/Prestige/Integrity

You may have noticed these symptoms in yourself or in others. The list of symptoms for someone with very strong Liver energy is as follows:

Physical Symptoms:

- Lung problems
- feeling of sadness/ depression
- Stomach/spleen problems (biggest)
- weak Heart function
- diabetes
- occasionally withdrawn due to weak Lung support
- lack of mental sharpness
- tiredness
- thyroid issues
- can't digest well
- negative thoughts
- lack of energy
- chest discomfort/pain
- Kidney/bladder issues
- rheumatism/arthritis

Behavioral Symptoms:

- not easily angered
- compassionate and considerate of others
- persistent but weak finish
- has difficulty entrusting any relationship issues to others
- stubborn
- loner
- indecisiveness
- disorderly
- inflexible
- slow but persistent
- kind
- intelligent
- collector
- religious
- thinks excessively
- obsessive and paranoid
- good memory system
- excellent planner
- good at nurturing and teaching
- weak sense of reality
- frugal

If these warning symptoms are ignored, depending on the condition of other organs, it will lead to Lung, Stomach, and Kidney problems.

*When this individual has suicidal thoughts, it indicates the depletion of his/her Lung energy. The Lung is basically dying out, unable to provide staying power to support the body system.

What will help ease the problem?

See "How to Improve My Health," Chapter 6

What's the benefit?

- more energy
- greater clarity
- open and upright chest
- more harmonious
- confident
- more independent
- better sleep

Strong Liver-Lung

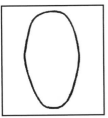

Each body organ exhibits characteristics unique to itself. This individual with strong Liver-Lung organs has major attachments/traits as follows:

Principled/Values integrity

You may have noticed these symptoms in yourself or in others. The list of symptoms for someone with strong Liver-Lung energy is as follows:

Physical Symptoms:

- Heart issues
- Kidney issues
- Kidney-related issues
- Stomach/spleen issues (biggest)
- overall, the body is weak
- hearing issues
- tiredness
- itching of the throat
- dry, stiff eyes
- artery blockage

Behavioral Symptoms:

- dominating/controlling
- natural leader
- precise judgment
- finishes strong despite appearing weak
- thinks excessively
- instability due to weak central grounding
- easily swayed (need caution)
- paranoid delusions
- no compassion

If you ignore these warning symptoms, it will lead to continued Stomach and spleen discomfort, and problems with the Kidneys, kidney stones, the reproductive organs, and the pancreas.

What will help ease the problem?

See "How to Improve My Health," Chapter 6

How will I benefit?

- calming of the lungs and the rest of the body
- more energy
- greater clarity
- focus
- fewer stomach issues
- improved colon health
- less demanding

Strong Liver-Stomach

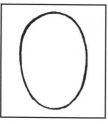

Each body organ exhibits characteristics unique to itself. This individual with strong Liver-Stomach organs has major attachments/traits as follows:

Gutsy/Knowledgeable/Acts dignified

You may have noticed these symptoms in yourself or in others. The list of symptoms for someone with strong Liver-Stomach energy is as follows:

Physical Symptoms:

- Heart issues
- Lung problems
- Kidney-related/bladder issues (biggest)
- thyroid issues
- rheumatism/arthritis
- hearing issues
- tiredness
- itching of the throat
- prostate issues
- poor blood/energy circulation
- artery blockage

Behavioral Symptoms:

- very devious
- very negative
- very gutsy
- smooth relationships with others
- into learning and research
- weak at finishing things except when it comes to money
- very passive/avoids clashing
- operates at slow/dull pace

If you ignore these warning symptoms, it will lead to continued Stomach and spleen discomfort, and problems with the Kidneys, kidney stones, the reproductive organs, and the pancreas.

What will help ease the problem?

See "How to Improve My Health," Chapter 6

How will I benefit?

- calm body
- more energy
- greater clarity
- focus
- fewer stomach issues
- more fair-minded

Strong Lungs

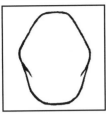

Each body organ exhibits characteristics unique to itself. This individual with strong Lung organ has major attachments/traits as follows:

Principled/Fair play/Being right

You may have noticed these symptoms in yourself or in others. The list of symptoms for someone with strong Lung energy is as follows:

Physical Symptoms:

- Stomach problems
- irregular heart beat
- reproductive issues
- bitter/burning taste of the mouth
- raised surface of the tongue

- hot flashes
- weak Liver/gallbladder (biggest/unable to control anger)
- darkening of the skin (when severe)
- smell of metal (when severe)

- constipation (burning sensation of anus when severe)
- chest pains (at times severe)
- tight muscles and joints
- tiredness
- cough has metallic sound

Behavioral Symptoms:

- sharp with criticism
- charismatic
- strong desire for power
- strong against strong opponent
- weak against weaker opponent
- unkind

- aggressive, like a bulldozer
- strong leader (like a general)
- a natural leader, always in command
- sharp thoughts
- quick decisions

- inconsiderate of others
- strongly opinionated
- no compassion for others
- believes in fair play
- independent thinker
- cool/cold personality
- keen eye
- stubborn

If these warning symptoms are ignored, depending on the condition of other organs, it will lead to Stomach, Heart, and Liver problems.

What will help ease the problem?

See "How to Improve My Health," Chapter 6

What's the benefit?

- more energy
- greater clarity
- more considerate
- calmer
- kind

- more harmonious
- less harsh words
- regular/happy bowel movements
- better sleep

Strong Lung-Kidney

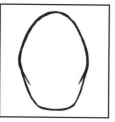 Each body organ exhibits characteristics unique to itself. This individual with strong Lung-Kidney organs has major attachments/traits as follows:

Principled/Independent decision maker

You may have noticed these symptoms in yourself or in others. The list of symptoms for someone with strong Lung-Kidney energy is as follows:

Physical Symptoms:

- sensitive colon
- Heart/small intestine issues (biggest)
- Stomach issues
- digestive problems
- chronic back problems
- skin issues
- joint stiffness
- catches cold easily
- vascular disease
- gets hot and cold
- weak esophagus
- slightly feverish at times
- unable to warm up easily
- tiredness
- shortness of breath

Behavioral Symptoms:

- lack of kindness
- rude
- cold personality
- blunt
- self-dignified
- anxiety
- opinionated
- impatient
- feeling of despondency/bleakness
- charismatic
- diligent
- intelligent
- rational
- loner tendency
- independent

If these warning symptoms are ignored, it will lead to continued Stomach dryness, spleen discomfort, Kidney, Heart, Stomach, and Liver problems.

What will help ease the problem?

See "How to Improve My Health," Chapter 6

What's the benefit?

- less back pain
- less cold
- a bit kinder
- more energy
- warmer
- less harsh towards oneself and others
- fewer stomach issues

Strong Lung-Heart

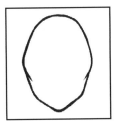

Each body organ exhibits characteristics unique to itself. This individual with strong Lung-Heart organs has major attachments/traits as follows:

Excellent investigator/ Able to see beyond the obvious

You may have noticed these symptoms in yourself or in others. The list of symptoms for someone with strong Lung-Heart energy is as follows:

Physical Symptoms:

- Kidney-related problems
- hot flashes
- Stomach problems
- weak Liver/gallbladder (biggest)
- tingling of fingers/toes
- leukemia
- constipation (burning sensation of anus when severe)
- tiredness at times
- lack of energy
- back issues
- tight muscles and joints

Behavioral Symptoms:

- impatient
- quick to anger
- big heart at times
- keen eye
- can appear cold/unkind but able to help others in different ways
- very strong focus
- acts like a military officer

If you ignore these warning symptoms and depending on the condition of your other organs, it can lead to major health crisis due to problems with the Stomach, Liver, and Kidney organs.

What will help ease the problem?

See How to Improve My Health (Chapter 6)

What's the benefit?

- fully energized
- wider clarity
- calm body
- regular and happy bowel movements
- better sleep
- feel more compassion toward others
- will shine brightly once the body is harmonized

Strong Lung-Liver

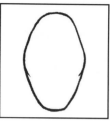

Each body organ exhibits characteristics unique to itself. This individual with strong Lung-Liver organs has major attachments/traits as follows:

Principled/Values integrity

You may have noticed these symptoms in yourself or in others. The list of symptoms for someone with strong Lung-Liver energy is as follows:

Physical Symptoms:

- Stomach/spleen issues (biggest)
- heart issues
- Kidney-related issues
- possible diabetes
- hearing issues
- tiredness
- itching of the throat
- artery blockage

Behavioral Symptoms:

- no compassion
- dominating
- controlling
- stubborn
- thinks excessively
- outgoing
- disciplined leader, like a bulldozer
- demanding
- power hungry/very spiritual

If you ignore these warning symptoms, it will lead to continued stomach and spleen discomfort, and problems with the Kidneys, kidney stones, the reproductive organs, and the pancreas.

What will help ease the problem?

See "How to Improve My Health," Chapter 6

What's the benefit?

- calming of the lungs and the rest of the body
- more energy
- greater clarity
- focus
- fewer stomach issues
- improved colon health
- less demanding

Strong Lung-Lung

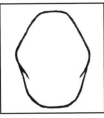

Each body organ exhibits characteristics unique to itself. This individual with very strong Lung organ has major attachments/traits as follows:

Principled/Fair play/Being right

You may have noticed these symptoms in yourself or in others. The list of symptoms for someone with very strong Lung energy is as follows:

Physical Symptoms:

- stomach problems
- irregular heart beat
- reproductive issues
- bitter/burning taste of the mouth
- raised surface of the tongue
- hot flashes (unable to control the system)
- leukemia
- uncontrollable anger (lacks Liver/gallbladder energy, the biggest issue)
- darkening of the skin (when severe)
- smell of metal (when severe)
- cough has metallic sound
- headache (lacks Liver energy)
- constipation/burning sensation of anus when severe (lacks Kidney energy)
- chest pains (at times severe)
- tight muscles and joints (lacks Kidney energy)
- tiredness
- artery blockage

Behavioral Symptoms:

- sharp with criticism
- charismatic
- strong desire for power
- strong against strong opponent while weak against weaker opponent
- unkind
- aggressive, like a bulldozer
- strong leader (like a general)
- a natural leader, always in command
- sharp thoughts
- stubborn
- inconsiderate of others
- strongly opinionated
- no compassion for others
- believe in fair play
- independent thinker
- "my way or no way" attitude
- very keen bird's eye point of view

If these warning symptoms are ignored, depending on the condition of other organs, it will lead to Stomach, Heart, and Liver problems.

What will help ease the problem?

See "How to Improve My Health," Chapter 6

What's the Benefit?

- more energy
- greater clarity
- more considerate
- calmer
- kind
- more harmonious
- fewer harsh words
- regular/happy bowel movements
- better sleep

Strong Lung-Stomach

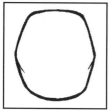

Each body organ exhibits characteristics unique to itself. This individual with strong Lung-Stomach organs has major attachments/traits as follows:

Domineering boss/ Pursuing education to gain knowledge

You may have noticed these symptoms in yourself or in others. The list of symptoms for someone with strong Lung-Stomach energy is as follows:

Physical Symptoms:

- sensitive colon
- irregular heart issues
- skin problems
- hearing issues
- feels slightly feverish
- at times feel elevated temperature
- tiredness
- poor eyesight

- tingling of fingers/ toes
- lower abdominal issues
- lack of fluid in the body system
- circulation problem
- artery blockage

- idle/stuck body system
- tightness of airways, blood vessels
- shortness of breath
- tight or itchy throat
- weak liver/gallbladder (biggest)
- weak muscle/tendon

Behavioral Symptoms:

- unkind
- impatient
- rude
- frugal
- perfectionist
- confident
- "know it all" attitude

- delusionally believes everyone to be beneath them
- unable to play truly fair-and-square
- poor circulation makes honesty difficult

- on quick impression seems bold/daring, but is actually devious
- appears weak and soft on the outside, but is strong and hard in the inside

If you ignore these warning symptoms, it will lead to Liver and gallbladder problems, continued Stomach dryness, spleen discomfort, and problems with the Kidneys, kidney stones, the reproductive organs, and the pancreas.

What will help ease the problem?

See "How to Improve My Health," Chapter 6

What's the benefit?

- more energy
- greater clarity
- better focus

- fewer stomach issues
- regular bowel movements

Strong Stomach

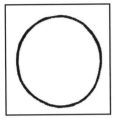

Each body organ exhibits characteristics unique to itself. This individual with strong Stomach organ has major attachments/traits as follows:

Charmer/Sweet talker/Hoarder of money/Desires longevity

You may have noticed these symptoms in yourself or in others. The list of symptoms for someone with very strong Stomach energy is as follows:

Physical Symptoms:

- dry lips and mouth
- dry skin
- dry stomach
- slight elevated body temperature
- lack of mental sharpness
- tingling of fingers and toes (extreme lack of Kidney energy)
- weak Kidney/bladder (biggest)
- hot flashes
- desire to lay down/sleep whenever possible
- uncomfortable body condition but unable to change it
- can't digest well
- easily tired
- feels like a balloon ready to pop
- constipation
- thyroid issues
- tightness of airways, blood vessels
- shortness of breath
- tight, itchy throat
- white coating on tongue
- sandy mouth feel
- tightness of ovaries, Kidneys
- urine feels hot/warm
- very weak lower body/like walking on clouds

Behavioral Symptoms:

- early bird
- diligent
- frugal
- warm
- devious
- arrogant/self-inflated
- extreme likes and dislikes
- not very talkative
- very negative
- inability to trust anyone with money issues
- indecisive
- practical
- shy of strangers

If these warning symptoms are ignored, depending on the condition of other organs, it will lead to Kidney failure, brain tumor, and problems with Stomach, thyroid, breast, reproductive organs, and pancreas.

What will help ease the problem?

See "How to Improve My Health," Chapter 6

What's the Benefit?

- cooler body temperature
- no more fog in the head
- clarity
- calm body
- softer skin
- regular/happy bowel movements
- better sleep

Strong Stomach-Kidney

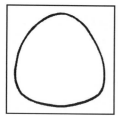

Each body organ exhibits characteristics unique to itself. This individual with strong Stomach-Kidney organs has major attachments/traits as follows:

Attracted to sunny people with strong heart energy/ Flows with the money

You may have noticed these symptoms in yourself or in others. The list of symptoms for someone with strong Stomach-Kidney energy is as follows:

Physical Symptoms:

- lack of energy
- breast issues
- very weak Heart function and small intestine (biggest)
- body often feels cold due to poor blood/energy circulation
- tiredness
- slow body function
- withdrawn at times
- urinary system issues
- venereal diseases

Behavioral Symptoms:

- very talkative, tries to dominate most conversations
- unkind opinions
- rude/unkind
- often anxious and unhappy
- lack of sincere appreciation
- unable to have a bubbly personality
- innovative
- calculating
- no warmth
- selfish/inconsiderate
- no compassion for others
- prone to negativity
- above normal appetite for sex and money
- a bit timid/shy
- extraordinary research skills
- tend to work in IT, research and science fields, and service industries

If these warning symptoms are ignored, depending on the condition of other organs, it will lead to Heart problems.

What will help ease the problem?

See "How to Improve My Health," Chapter 6

What's the Benefit?

- more energy
- greater clarity
- a calm body
- more considerate
- warm and stable
- look younger
- regular and happy bowel movements
- better sleep

Strong Stomach-Heart

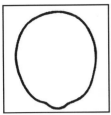

Each body organ exhibits characteristics unique to itself. This individual with strong Stomach-Heart organs has major attachments/traits as follows:

Money/Beauty/Greed

You may have noticed these symptoms in yourself or in others. The list of symptoms for someone with strong Stomach-Heart energy is as follows:

Physical Symptoms:

- dry lips and skin
- dry Stomach
- can't digest well
- constipation
- forgets easily
- depression
- body discomfort
- lack of mental sharpness
- feels like an inflating balloon, ready to pop
- slightly elevated body temperature
- slight fever (inside body)
- hot flashes
- desire to lay down/sleep
- body feels lazy but is able to go shopping
- easily tired except when at the center of attention
- diabetes
- thyroid issues
- tightness of airways, blood vessels
- shortness of breath
- tight, itchy throat
- tightness of ovaries, Kidneys
- discomfort while urinating
- air bubble in urine
- Kidney/bladder issues (biggest issue)

Behavioral Symptoms:

- prone to suicidal thoughts
- natural artist
- entertainer
- witty
- nonconventional
- circumspect/prudent
- weak at finishing tasks/things
- weak at managing finances
- strong focus/obsession with money/finances (for spending)
- diligent
- bright on the outside, negative in the inside

If these warning symptoms are ignored, depending on the condition of other organs, it will lead to brain tumor, and thyroid, breast, reproductive, and pancreatic problems.

What will help ease the problem?

See "How to Improve My Health," Chapter 6

What's the Benefit?

- body cools down
- clarity
- calms the body
- better sleep
- softer skin
- regular and happy bowel movements

Strong Stomach-Liver

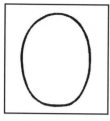

Each body organ exhibits characteristics unique to itself. This individual with strong Stomach-Liver organs has major attachments/traits as follows:

Domineering boss/Pursuit of education

You may have noticed these symptoms in yourself or in others. The list of symptoms for someone with strong Stomach-Liver energy is as follows:

Physical Symptoms:

- sensitive colon
- irregular Heart issues
- skin problems
- at times feel elevated temperature
- hearing issues
- artery blockage

- Kidney, bladder, and hormonal issues (biggest issues)
- lack of fluid in the body system
- circulation problems

- idle/stuck body system
- tiredness
- tightness of airways, blood vessels
- shortness of breath
- tight or itchy throat
- thyroid issues

Behavioral Symptoms:

- lack of kindness (inside)
- intelligent
- diligent
- passive nature
- very negative thoughts

- unable to play truly fair-and-square
- traditional/conservative
- gets along with others

If you ignore these warning symptoms, it will lead to continued Stomach dryness, spleen discomfort, and problems with the Kidneys, kidney stones, the reproductive organs, and the pancreas.

What will help ease the problem?

See "How to Improve My Health," Chapter 6

How will I benefit?

- more energy
- greater clarity
- focus
- fewer stomach issues
- regular bowel movements

Strong Stomach-Lung

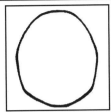

Each body organ exhibits characteristics unique to itself. This individual with strong Stomach-Lung organs has major attachments/traits as follows:

Frugal businessperson/Quietly works to accumulate wealth

You may have noticed these symptoms in yourself or in others. The list of symptoms for someone with strong Stomach-Lung energy is as follows:

Physical Symptoms:

- skin problems
- hearing issues
- tiredness
- shortness of breath
- tight or itchy throat
- weak muscles/ tendons
- artery blockage

- irregular Heart issues
- feels slightly feverish
- at times feel elevated temperature
- tingling of fingers/ toes
- lower abdominal issues

- lack of fluid in the body system
- circulation problem
- idle/stuck body system
- tightness of airways, blood vessels
- tight or itchy throat
- Liver/gallbladder issues

Behavioral Symptoms:

- delusionally believes everyone to be beneath them
- unkind
- impatient
- rude
- frugal
- wears modest clothing
- "know it all" attitude

- confident
- independent
- curiosity for new things
- appears soft and weak on the outside, but is strong and hardened on the inside

- poor circulation makes honesty difficult
- on quick impression seems bold/daring, but is actually devious
- plays to win only for him/ herself while giving others crumbs to convince them of how "fair" he/she is

If you ignore these warning symptoms, it will lead to continued Stomach dryness, spleen discomfort, and problems with the Kidneys, kidney stones, the reproductive organs, and the pancreas.

What will help ease the problem?

See "How to Improve My Health," Chapter 6

How will I benefit?

- more energy
- greater clarity
- focus
- fewer stomach issues
- regular bowel movements

Strong Stomach-Stomach

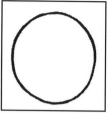

Each body organ exhibits characteristics unique to itself. This individual with very strong Stomach organ has major attachments/traits as follows:

Collector/Hoarding money/Desire for longevity

You may have noticed these symptoms in yourself or in others. The list of symptoms for someone with very strong Stomach energy is as follows:

Physical Symptoms:

- dry lips and mouth
- dry skin
- dry Stomach
- slight elevated body temperature
- lack of mental sharpness
- hot flashes
- Liver/Kidney issues (biggest issue)
- Heart issue
- constipation
- artery blockage

- desire to lay down/sleep whenever possible
- uncomfortable body condition but unable to change it
- can't digest well
- easily tired
- feels like a balloon ready to pop
- poor circulation
- feel cold
- thyroid issues

- tightness of airways, blood vessels
- shortness of breath
- tight, itchy throat
- white coating on tongue
- sandy mouth feel
- tightness of ovaries, Kidneys
- urine feels hot/warm (bladder issue)
- prostate issue
- diabetes

Behavioral Symptoms:

- tries to be confident
- very frugal, some cases very extravagant
- very warm and friendly

- inability to trust anyone with money issues
- internally very negative due to lack of kidney support

- early bird
- diligent
- frugal
- stubborn

If these warning symptoms are ignored, depending on the condition of other organs, it will lead to Kidney failure, brain tumor, and problems with Stomach, thyroid, breast, reproductive organs, and pancreas.

What will help ease the problem?

See "How to Improve My Health," Chapter 6

What's the Benefit?

- cooler body temperature
- no more fog in the head
- clarity

- calm body
- softer skin
- regular/happy bowel movements
- better sleep

Chapter 4

Food for the Organs

Food Summary

Some of us went through food shortages in the distant past where we had to eat anything and everything to survive. We couldn't be picky. We ate what we could, and when we could, just to survive from day to day.

And some of us had abundance of food to choose from. Despite that, we ate only certain foods that were embedded into our system by our choices/habits. If we were going to eat, why not eat whatever we wanted? We could keep eating all kinds of food that didn't agree with us until our body was no longer able to support it.

From these experiences we acquired certain food tastes and habits that remained with us even after decades and centuries have passed. And from time to time, a memory of a certain food pops up in our head. Why? The dominant organ in our body wants that food to imbalance the system. Without realizing this, we try the food. At first, it seems to give us comfort and pleasure, but then discomfort begins to emerge. Soon, it's not comfort food anymore and we remember why we no longer ate that food.

Although some places still suffer from food insecurity, many of us have the luxury of choosing what to eat, how much to eat, and how often to eat it. We have many more ways with which to supply our body with food. Some are beneficial to our body system while others make us sick.

Sometimes we rely on our sense of taste, sound, smell, sight and touch in choosing what we eat. They aren't always the correct guide in choosing what is good for us. The senses are only interpreting what is before them and we blindly follow. And without realizing, we eat the foods that make us sick on a continual basis. It feels like comfort food for some, while for others it's habit food.

From time to time, we realize that a particular food makes us sick and we decide to avoid it in the future. At the beginning of this realization we remember to avoid the food. But soon, we forget and seek the food that made us sick in the first place. The damaging food might be pulling us from our past eating habits, or because one of our strong organs desires more power, which damages the rest of the organ systems. The program just keeps running and running.

The only way to stop the automatic programming from the past is to realize what is going on now, in our present moment. We have to decide whether to continue with the old programming that makes us sick, or to amend the program by changing into new habits that are based on a new way of looking at and consuming food.

Our initial response to the food list may be one of the following:

"Oh, that's good. I'm already eating most of the items on this list. I will need to make only a few changes."

At this point we may need only a bit of adjustment to attain better health, money, power, dignity, and longevity.

"I don't have any of those food items in my food pantry or the refrigerator. It's going to cost me an up-front investment for myself and my family."

Following the list and becoming healthy actually saves money. When we continue to eat foods that aren't good for us, the food we spent our money on simply sits in our stomach, creating indigestion, heartburn, constipation, poor circulation, etc. And whatever food doesn't get distributed to the organs gets flushed down the toilet, which is money down the toilet. That food serves no other purpose than to fill our stomach, while creating havoc for our body system as it works to rid itself of it. When we do this over and over again, we create continual suffering for ourselves. If we actually eat what is beneficial for us, the money spent on that food is not wasted.

"What is there for me to eat? The list shows none of the foods that I like."

The body has been supplied with the wrong foods. For a while, it may be okay, as the body does what it can to make ends meet. But eventually, the body will run out of ways to support itself. What then? We can look for a miracle to fix the problem. And even if a miracle does happen, do we change? No, we keep on neglecting our body until there is nothing left at the end.

The battle within ourselves will be long and hard because the organ system is so off balance, with one or two dominating the other organs. Reaching the middle ground for the body to balance itself will take time, unless we decide to make dramatic improvements right now to get there faster.

Eating what our body needs is more economical, less time consuming, less stressful, and will ultimately save us money by not having to remedy the damage done by poor eating habits.

When selecting food items, the first choice will be fresh and naturally ripened food.

If fresh isn't available, our second choice will be frozen foods, and then dried foods as our third choice. Be sure to choose quality foods that are nontoxic because our body will return the favor by providing us with the energy we need to function more efficiently.

Which food gives us more power to our systems?

We often believe that animal protein gives us greater power. In reality, some naturally grown raw grains provide six times greater energy power than meat. Ironically, we feed the grain to our animals instead of eating it ourselves. Why?

The rich nutrients of the grains never really reach us because that's not what the animals naturally eat. The cows, for example, were designed to eat grass, but we feed them grains, which they can't fully digest and transfer to us. We should just directly eat the grains ourselves instead of trying to get it through the animals we eat. For the animals, they benefit from being consumed by humans because it gives them a chance to get closer to the human realm. We, on the other hand, will be kept from reaching higher levels due to the heaviness of animal habits and traits that get embedded into our body system through what we eat.

If we eat animal meat on a regular basis rather than for medicinal purposes, we will end up with a heavy accumulation of animal traits and energies if we don't know how to remove them regularly from our body system.

Cooked or raw food?

Cooked foods often taste better and are easier to eat, but they provide us with only 20%–30% of its original nutritional value. Unsatisfied, we end up eating other things in our attempt to fill our body's nutritional needs.

Fresh or dry, raw foods have a lot of flavor, but they may not suit our taste due to the lack of usual seasonings. But when we consume raw fresh uncooked food, 90%–100% of its nutritional value gets delivered to our body, so we can stay healthy even with only a small portion. There is no need to overload our body and we can extend our life span in the process.

Once we decide to take care of our body with both cooked and raw foods, and be responsible owners of it, we may be surprised by how well our body begins to function.

Food is a necessary and powerful tool for staying healthy. What we eat daily affects how we feel physically, mentally, emotionally, and spiritually.

Kidney Foods for Weak Kidneys

Consuming these food items will strengthen the Kidneys. The strongest energy items are listed at the beginning. *Those with diatheses such as food sensitivity/ allergies should check ingredients before taking.*

Grains	barley, buckwheat, farro wheat (spelt), black rice
Beans	black beans (the tiny ones), adzuki
Nuts	most nuts okay
Seeds	black sesame
Veggies	bamboo shoots, cucumber, mung bean sprouts, beets, cilantro, celery, zucchini, mushrooms, asparagus, (non-bitter) lettuce, savory, chicory, radishes, bitter melon, jicama, watercress, iceberg lettuce
Neutral Veggies	broccoli, cauliflower, kale, lettuce, onions, parsley, bell peppers
Fruits	cranberry, lychee, watermelon, durian, kiwi, Korean pear, Asian pear, pomegranates, honeydew melon, raspberry, strawberry, blackberry, coconut
Meats	pork, bone marrow, bone broth (stock)
Seafoods	sea cucumber, sea squirt, edible seaweeds (kelp, bladder wrack, sea grapes, chlorella, etc.), octopus, mussels, shrimp
Seasoning	bamboo salt neutral: miso, soy sauce, salt (in moderation)
Oil	coconut oil, black sesame seed oil okay with canola, corn, nut oils, olive, peanut, safflower, sesame, soybean, sunflower, veggie
Spreads	N/A
Beverages Teas	cranberry juice, aloe vera juice, teas (black, oolong, Earl Grey, English breakfast), bitter melon, barley
Alcohol	beer
Sweeteners	N/A
Misc. Items	cheese, echinacea/golden seal, licorice, cordyceps mushroom

Heart Foods for the Weak Heart

Consuming these food items will strengthen the Heart. The strongest energy items are listed at the beginning. *An asterisk indicates indirect benefit. Those with diatheses such as food sensitivity/allergies should check ingredients before taking.*

Grains	corn, Indian millet, teff, red sorghum, foxtail millet wild rice*
Beans	pinto
Nuts	most nuts okay
Seeds	sunflower, sesame, pumpkin seeds
Veggies	(anything that tastes bitter) radicchio/Italian lettuce, eggplant, lotus root, carrot, tomato, Brussels sprouts, cabbage, dandelion, mugwort, endive, bell flower root, codonopsis, dried mushrooms, tomatillo
Neutral Veggies	broccoli, cauliflower, kale, lettuce, onions, parsley, bell peppers
Fruits	mangosteen, apricot, grapefruit, banana, plantains, passion fruit
Meats	lamb, duck, quail, chicken, turkey, veal, venison
Seafoods	squid, yellow dried pollack (Hwangtae)
Seasoning	cooking wine, jjajang sauce/Korean black bean paste
Oil	extra virgin olive, sunflower, okay with canola, corn, nut oils, peanut, safflower, sesame, soybeans, veggie
Spreads	chocolate spreads, chocolate-related sweets
Beverages Teas	coffee, corn tea, ginseng, cocoa, green tea, mocha, dandelion tea, bellflower root tea, chaga tea
Alcohol	sake, rum, gin, vodka, soju, brandy, sherry
Sweeteners	N/A
Misc. Items	ginseng, 100% dark chocolate, echinacea/golden seal, reishi mushroom, chaga mushroom, shitake mushroom, yogurt, omega 3-6-9 oil

Liver Foods for the Weak Liver

Consuming these food items will strengthen the Liver. The strongest energy items are listed at the beginning. *An asterisk indicates indirect benefit. Those with diatheses such as food sensitivity/allergies should check ingredients before taking.*

Grains	alfalfa, quinoa, wheat, oat, rye, bulgur, lentils
Beans	all beans except the adzuki and the tiny black bean
Nuts	most nuts (except for almonds and pine nuts)
Seeds	perilla, sesame, pumpkin, sunflower,
Veggies	all leafy greens, artichoke, okra, bean sprout, arrowroot, avocado, olive, kale, broccoli
Neutral Veggies	broccoli, cauliflower, kale, lettuce, onions, parsley, bell peppers
Fruits	green apple, apples, blueberry, huckleberry, lemon, lime, kiwi, tangerine, elderberry, grapes, oranges, pomegranate, plums, prunes, most berries, raisins
Meats	chicken, eggs, quail, turkey
Seafoods	all clams (except for abalone, scallops and other shell fish), clam juice
Seasoning	miso, vinegar
Oil	canola, corn, nut oils, extra virgin olive, peanut, safflower, sesame, soybeans, sunflower, perilla, grapeseed
Spreads	apple butter, sesame butter, plum, peanut butter, mayonnaise
Beverages Teas	sesame, omija tea, apple, orange, grape, plum, prune juice, soy milk
Alcohol	wine, fruit coolers
Sweeteners	okay with brown sugar,* carob, chocolate,* corn syrup,* honey,* maple syrup,* molasses, rice syrup/rice malt, sucanat, white sugar
Misc. Items	Susin Ogapy Royal (*acanthopanax koreanum*), flax seed oil, omega 3-6-9 oil, sour tastes/vitamin C, echinacea/golden seal, protein powder, soft tofu, soy products

Lung Foods For Weak Lungs

Consuming these food items will strengthen the Lungs. The strongest energy items are listed at the beginning. *An asterisk indicates indirect benefit. Those with diatheses such as food sensitivity/allergies should check ingredients before taking.*

Grains	brown rice, pearl barley, chia
Beans	all beans are beneficial
Nuts	pine nuts, almonds, gingko nuts
Seeds	mustard, mustard green seeds, radish seeds
Veggies	all turnip family, mustard green, mustard, garlic, chives, green onions, ginger, turmeric, radish, sage, arugula, coriander, marjoram, cumin, thyme, bay leaves, rosemary, basil, napa cabbage, perilla leaf, chard, onions, parsnips, rutabaga, scallion, fennel, bok choy
Neutral Veggies	broccoli, cauliflower, kale, lettuce, onions, parsley, bell peppers
Fruits	Korean pear, currants, peach, pineapple, banana, nectarine, pear cactus (fragosika), dragon fruit (pitaya), jack fruit
Meats	fish, beef (beef consumption is for medicinal purpose. Take only for a short time because the beef's toxic heaviness remains in our body system for 3–7 days or longer, depending on the body type.)
Seafoods	all seafoods except for squid and octopus
Seasoning	chili pepper, black pepper, white pepper, dill, all spices
Oil	mustard seed, safflower, red chili-pepper oil okay with canola, corn, nut oils, olive, peanut, safflower, sesame, soybean, sunflower, veggie
Spreads	almond butter, butter
Beverages Teas	mint tea, pineapple, pear (Korean pear), milk, almond milk, chamomile tea, pearl barley tea
Alcohol	N/A
Sweeteners	okay with brown sugar, carob, chocolate,* corn syrup,* honey,* molasses, rice syrup/rice malt, sucanat
Misc. Items	gingko, aloe vera juice, echinacea/golden seal, high quality fish oil, all dairy products

Food for the Organs

Stomach Foods for the Weak Stomach

Consuming these food items will strengthen the Stomach. The strongest energy items are listed at the beginning. *An asterisk indicates indirect benefit. Those with diatheses such as food sensitivity/allergies should check ingredients before taking.*

Grains	sweet rice, corn, white rice, wild rice, proso millet, sorghum
Beans	lima,* navy,* pinto,* soy,* kidney*
Nuts	cashews, peanuts
Seeds	okay with sesame, pumpkin, sunflower
Veggies	spinach, cabbage, lotus root, carrot, potatoes, sweet potatoes, yams, winter squash, parsnip, jicama, butternut squash
Neutral Veggies	broccoli, cauliflower, kale, lettuce, onions, parsley, bell peppers
Fruits	dates, figs, mangos, papaya, American pears, cantaloupe, banana
Meats	N/A
Seafoods	N/A
Seasoning	cinnamon, ginger, honey, brown sugar
Oil	okay with canola, corn, nut oils, olive, safflower, sesame, soybean, sunflower, veggie
Spreads	N/A
Beverages Teas	pu'erh tea, corn tea, ginger tea, ginseng, Chinese yam tea, jujube tea, mango juice, goji tea
Alcohol	brandy,* fruit coolers,* gin,* rum,* sake,* sherry,* wine,* vodka*
Sweeteners	carob, corn syrup,* honey, maple syrup,* molasses, rice syrup/rice malt, sucanat, white sugar
Misc. Items	propolis, royal jelly, echinacea/golden seal, wild raw honey, tapioca

Knowing How Much to Eat and When to Stop

How do I know if I ate the wrong food or too much of something?

Our Stomach communicates to us through burping when we eat too much of something or the wrong food for our body. We can sometimes taste the food sitting in our Stomach, not taken by the other organs. If the food is the correct type for our body but we burp, then what the body is telling us is that we ate in excess, with no organs needing them at the current time.

What happens when I discontinue following the food list?

We will slowly go back to where we started.

How long will my condition last once I stop eating these recommended foods?

It all depends on how much we've accumulated and how our body is utilizing it. But it will return to where it was rather quickly.

How long will it take for my body to correct itself?

We won't know until we've reached it. When we reach that point, we will know. Our system will record all our endeavors, and we will be able to access the information in the future. This is a good investment for better health and mental clarity.

Can I recommend my diet to others?

We must not recommend our foods to others, as they may not have the exact organ system as we have. In the long term, it may be more harmful than beneficial for them.

Right food items and right amounts?

Many of us may not have eaten the food items needed by our organs and are wondering if we are eating enough of the right foods.

When it comes to the correct organ food for our body, when the body has had enough of it, we will feel content and stop eating. There is no searching for more of it because our body is satisfied with what has been provided.

If our body is still hungry for more of something, experiment through our category of food items. We haven't provided what our body system needs yet.

Once we provide our body with what it needs and reach satisfaction and balance, we will be good for a while. We save ourselves from eating this and that for no particular benefit and save a lot of money in the process. And we will become calmer than ever before.

What to avoid eating first thing in the morning on an empty stomach?

For most of us, our body structures can't handle it when we eat sweet foods first in the morning, on an empty stomach. We have been told how an apple a day will keep the doctor away. However, if those of us who have weak Stomach eat an apple as the first thing each morning, it will be a very different story. That apple, upon entering the empty stomach, will create excess acid and agitate the stomach wall. This in turn will plunge the body into an emergency shock mode until the body system sufficiently recovers from the distress. We need to understand that for some of us, our body system can only tolerate this for a short time.

However, what if we have a very strong Stomach and eat an apple first thing in the morning because we've been told that it's good for us? In this case, our body system will divert all of the liquid from the other organs and send it to the Stomach. If we continue this habit without supplying sufficient Kidney energy to our body system, we will encounter serious health issues and Kidney-related problems such as kidney stones, thyroid issues, circulation problems, diabetes, muscle and joint issues, fatigue, teeth problems, and so on.

Sometimes, what is supposed to be good for us is simply wrong for our body type. If we have a strong Lung body structure and eat tomatoes on an empty stomach at the beginning of the day because it's supposed to be good for us, we won't be functioning well due to excess acidity created by the tomato. Our body becomes agitated and unhappy because it is the wrong food for this body structure. However, for other body structures, tomatoes can be beneficial.

All of us are built differently with different combinations of organ energy strengths. It is essential that we listen to our body signals and work with our body system when eating the foods that are supposed to be good for us. Ultimately, it is our body that will tell us whether the food is beneficial or not.

No matter how good certain food items may be for us, we must know when to eat and when not to eat them. If we eat certain beneficial foods at the wrong time, or in the wrong sequence, they won't do much for us other than to create problems. If some of the food items aren't working for our body structure, let's not argue with logic. Our logic won't be able to change any of our body's problems. Simply avoid the food, or find another way to eat it without causing unnecessary harm.

Our body has told us many times that the troubling foods aren't working for us. How much damage do we need to inflict on ourselves before finally listening to what our body is telling us and becoming free from our agonies?

Let's learn to know what works and doesn't for our body system, and make adjustments accordingly.

Chapter 5

DNA

Why Did I Get the Short End
of the Stick in Life?

No matter that we got the short end of the stick or the long end of the stick, we are simply playing out what is in our DNA. It can be something that was just recorded or something that was stored from a distant past. Regardless, it decides who we are, how we live, how we think, who we partner with, what profession we choose, what we like or dislike, and even how we die. Until we realize this and desire to make changes, we will live into the continuum the life that we have programmed and recorded into our DNA.

Whether we are healthy, wealthy, famous, powerful, dignified, blessed with longevity, good, bad, or ugly, all outcomes are stored within us consciously or unconsciously. Since this is what we have recorded, this is what will play out accordingly in our life.

The good news is that since we were able to input, we are also able to amend and make updates as we see fit, thus changing the outcome. For permanent changes, we have to have a wake-up call or genuine realizations.

Some people are able to make small steps while others are able to make giant leaps. It is up to the individual.

What are the qualifications to being healthy?

In order to be healthy, we need to take care of the organ system, so it can function properly. We must adjust and balance the health of all organs so they are supporting each other instead of having one trying to dominate the other. And mental directing may seem to work at first but ultimately the method will not work as we hope. It happens only through true understanding/realizations. When our body reaches a certain comfort level, we begin to see or realize things. (*See* "How to Improve My Health," Chapter 6.)

What are the qualifications to being wealthy?

The organ system that is good at making money and knows money must first be strengthened. And we must strengthen the organ system that is able to hold onto that wealth. Each organ body system requires strengthening of different organs. (*See* "How to Improve Health, Money, Dignity and Longevity," Chapter 8.)

If those organs are fragile, we can't make this happen. We must first enhance the organs that will allow the money to stay and be secure in the storage. We must know our body and take care of it.

I don't know anything about DNA or stored information.

All our accumulated deeds, actions, and knowledge are stored in our DNA system and will generate output when the time comes. Some might ask, "How do I know that it's in my system?"

We access it all the time. We just don't know what to call it. Or, we may simply want to deny it and not acknowledge it, hoping that it will go away. But we are certain to follow or do certain things better than others and sometimes be surprised that we are able to know or do things without having learned to do them in this life.

It is like the child who plays a musical instrument without any lessons or having seen anyone do it, and insists on being a musician. That is the child's dream and he/she achieves it because of the previous knowledge/habits that's been stored and is playing out without any new learning. It's all stored in the child's DNA.

It's also like the child who wants to be a doctor even though none in his family is in the medical field. And so on, and so on. We do this all the time, living out our present moments with the information stored from our past.

Take my father for example, who ate fish all his life. He ate it every day without fail. He ate other things at a very minimum out of courtesy to the people serving him the food. But his focus was fish. Even at that, he ate only small portions during each meal and a little bit of beef broth from time to time. He only ate certain fruits and only a small amount at a time. After each meal, he would smoke a third of a single cigarette.

That was not considered a healthy diet or recommended as a standard diet for anyone. But that's what he ate all his life. He was healthy for most of his life and lived to 90 years of age while most of his friends died in their 60s or 70s. His friends told him to eat all kinds of good and exotic foods that would make him look good until the day he died. He just smiled and didn't take anyone's opinion when it came to his diet. He simply continued on with his regimen.

I didn't ask him why he did what he did and where he had learned to do that.

And he never offered the secret to me. But he continued on until three days before his death.

I don't eat fish. I don't even like the smell of fish cooking. It upsets my stomach. His wife didn't like the smell of fish cooking either, but she cooked fish every day for him for almost seven decades. She would ask, "Don't you ever get sick of fish?" He would smile and say, "That fish makes me feel centered and fulfilled for some reason." He only ate small portions everyday but he was healthy, outgoing, and popular in the town, city, and county where he lived. He invited VIPs and entertained them five to ten times a year. They were big group gatherings, yet he tried to maintain his eating habits. It was interesting to see when people offered food to him that he didn't normally eat. He would gently refuse and if they continued to insist, he would accept and put it on his plate, telling them he would eat it later. He maintained his eating ritual no matter what.

His mind was sharp. How sharp? Three days before his passing, he informed his wife that he must prepare for his earthly departure. He wouldn't be taking in any food. He had to empty what was in his system for his departure to the other world.

Later, I learned that he was one of the few rare individuals who knew what foods he had to eat to have his body function better. The specific foods that he had consumed every day of his life had represented his health, money, dignity, and longevity. He had lacked them in his body system.

No matter what's presently written in our DNA, we can still update/improve our health and more by simply changing our thoughts and eating habits.

How do people know and follow it?

Knowing and following their knowing is so natural for some it's as if it were cemented into their DNA, while it's not so natural for others.

For some, it can be as simple as the weather or the changing seasons.

When spring approaches us, we feel good. After having spent long cold months of winter, we look forward to stretching our bodies in the warm spring energy ahead. And as spring temperatures heat up, we shed our heavy clothing.

And when summer comes, we shed even more clothing and dress lightly. We don't insist on wearing our winter clothes, do we?

When fall comes, we put away the summer clothing.

When winter comes, we put on our heavy clothing to protect us from the cold.

We do these things naturally, without having anyone tell us when, what or how to do it. That is unless we have a malfunctioning signal system.

We may have noticed that some people are still in their summer shorts even in winter. While most of us are unable to comfortably spend winter in summer clothes, there are some who possess a body system that is strong enough to withstand the winter cold without any heavy clothing. It's not something a person with a weak body system should try to emulate, because that body won't be able to handle it and will get sick quickly.

It's that simple and obvious, but we refuse to acknowledge our individual body's weather. All we have to do is pay attention and see what our body needs. We use our body every second of our lives. Though we've received some education on how to take care of our body, it's not enough to attend to all of our body's needs. It's our responsibility to know, understand, and take care of our body as much as possible.

Some people have a body system with Spring temperature.

Some people have a body system with Summer temperature.

Some people have a body system with Fall temperature.

Some people have a body system with Winter temperature.

Some people have a body system with between-seasons temperature.

Some people have a body system with myriad seasonal temperatures.

Know the difference and take care of the body accordingly.

It's that simple.

How do our organs know which foods to take and which foods to avoid?

We don't give our body the proper credit it deserves, nor acknowledge the built-in capacity and functions of our organs. Each organ comes with specifications. With a car, one section requires water while another requires oil for its maintenance. Though these two sections serve two different purposes, they work together to run the entire car. This is the part that we must understand.

Once we know where the water and the oil goes, and understand the functional operation of Forward, Reverse, Neutral, and so on, we can maintain and drive the car properly.

For our body, we take almost everything through the mouth. The stomach chews and filters what we consume and then distributes it to each organ, if all the parts are in working condition. When individual organs become weak and low on energy, they wait for the delivery of the food that they need. And when we supply them with what they need (*see* How to Improve My Health, Chapter 6), we experience the receipt of the food that was delivered directly to the intended organs. We experience this without question.

If one of our organs or parts is not working properly, the food for that organ will sit in the stomach and later release out of the system as waste. Our body's organ system is far more advanced than we give it credit for.

It would save us from so much suffering if we just recognized the important and necessary purpose and functions of our internal organs. Without understanding our own body's manual, we create a lot of unnecessary hardship in our lives.

Did I Always Have This Puzzling DNA?

It's an information storehouse of acquired habits and traits, where our changing thoughts modify our behavior and get encoded into our DNA, altering our information system. It is through this system that we learn what's important for us to remember and live by. Some things we let go of based on what we want and desire, and so on, bringing us to our current condition.

Most of us depend on experts to tell us what is good for us and what is not. Sometimes it works and sometimes it doesn't. And sometimes, we consult them with normal maintenance issues that we ourselves should be responsible for. It's important to do our part by understanding and maintaining our body first, and then consult with experts for things that we lack knowledge in. This way, the experts can go beyond their current capacity to better serve us in the future, and we can more consciously evolve as we live out our lives.

Why do I have to learn and know this?

Because this is our body, it's our responsibility as owners to take care of it. And we don't want unnecessary suffering. How will a broken body take us where we want to go?

If we don't know our body system, we won't know what is true or not. We are at the mercy of someone who knows how to manipulate this situation for their own gains. If others have the upper hand over our body systems, we will be subject to slavery or be led astray without realizing it. It's important to ponder where we are with our own information.

How long do I need to continue taking care of my body system?

We have to nurture our body so that we can do things as a healthy person and develop better traits to carry with us into the future. Appreciate and take good care of it until the end, being a good, kind, and nurturing owner. All our habits and traits will be carried over to the next life and will resume uninterrupted. Though we will have a new body, the information will remain the same as we continue where we left off. For better or worse, we are the result of our actions with no one else to blame. Whatever we have recorded into our DNA will continue to remain until we consciously choose to make corrections in order to improve/evolve as human beings.

Can I blame someone for my imperfect DNA?

Yes. We can certainly do that. However, it comes right back to us. Instead of fruitless blaming, let's bear tangible fruit by improving ourselves and our situation.

The earth is the training ground on which we learn, upgrade, and evolve to the next level. If we aren't satisfied with taking one step at a time, then we can take a giant leap by realizing through awareness, and wake up from the dream within a dream.

I don't like what I have. Can I change it?

Yes. When we genuinely recognize the need for change within ourselves, then we can make deliberate changes. But just wishing won't make it so. Any need for change must come through true realizations.

It is also imperative that the organ system is secured. This means that there are no weak organs in the system. When our organ system is secured and healthy, no matter what comes our way to disturb our life, we can make it through without panic and fear. Often, it is panic and fear that prevent us from making the right decisions.

As it is our responsibility, let us understand ourselves and fill the holes and then step up into the major league of life. What if our innate gifts and talents aren't allowed to flourish and bear fruit because we don't understand our own body system? What if our potential to become the greatest teacher, nurse, wife, husband, doctor, lawyer, artist, actor, scientist, senator, or president of the world goes unfulfilled all because we forgot to take care of our foundation, our health?

Without securing our health base, we are sitting ducks when dealing with pain, agony, and confusion. From this place we pray to our God. Sometimes prayers are answered without us doing anything. And sometimes, the answer comes as an instruction on how to get out of the situation we're in. Oftentimes, we refuse to understand the instructions because we are hoping for a miracle that requires us to do nothing. It is possible, but we need to first upgrade ourselves to that level. Until then, from this physical realm, we may be required to follow instructions to get us out of the difficulties of this earthly existence. It is our responsibility to make this happen. We've been gifted with tremendous power that resides within us, so let us be wise and be responsible for ourselves.

The Energies at Birth

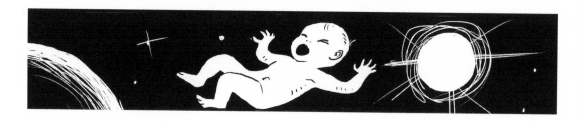

At birth, we bring with us all the stored information and transfer it into our new body. Some may add or some may exclude a few items for this life's endeavor if it is a birth with a special purpose.

When we come out of our mother's womb, the umbilical cord is cut and we take our first breath. We either cry or yawn, taking in whatever energy the universe provides at the time. This determines the strength of each of our organs and the organs' energy systems. It will decide whether we will have a strong kidney, heart, liver, lung, stomach and other connecting organs, and the strength of these organs will determine how our physical body functions.

To be clear, we are only talking about the physical part of ourselves.

It's rare for one to be born with a harmonized energy body structure. Most of us are not harmonized. And without fail, we will live out our lives exactly according to the way we are built. We do this in spite of our natural design that still allows us to grow and make improvements upon it if we so desire. A small portion of the population is not affected as much by their condition, but most of us live out our non-harmonized system. We must take care of our body to reach our full capacity and, through this, learn to amend and upgrade ourselves. However, we are often stuck in one particular thought or place and so, we have much to evolve.

To balance the body, we must feed the parts that are the weakest to help create balance within. And when necessary, trim the strong parts down. However, if we have a specific task in our lives that must be accomplished, one that requires that particular strong organ energy, then we shouldn't change anything until the task is done. We can harmonize afterwards. Often though, we continue in our old lifestyle even though we have done the required work. We must be aware of the different roles each organ plays in our lives in order to accomplish our life's goal, and evolve into the next continuum.

How Do I Change My Internal Information That I Do Not Like?

Changes are very simple.

If we make a realization or discover the need for change, we make the changes through *doing*. New inputs through real actions will override the old stored information.

However, if we "change" only through our thoughts or fantasies, the old information will remain active and continue to spin without a clear destination until we have actually performed the changes. We must put our realizations into actions.

Sometimes it is easy to do this work and other times it feels impossible no matter how much I try. Why is this?

When we have a somewhat harmonized internal organ system and a proper virtue account in place (*see* "Virtue Account," Chapter 9), it is easy to make this happen. All the organs are able to understand the signals and are in agreement with the need to cooperate with our intentions.

When we have deficiencies in some of our organs, or are lacking in our virtue account, it is difficult to make the changes. There is no energy for us to work with. Without all of the organs' participation and support, we are unable to make things happen as we hope. The first thing is to fill the deficiencies and then work on the changes. A broken wheel can't take us where we need to go.

And there are times when it feels like we can't fill the gaps in our system fast enough. When this happens, we do our best to maintain the harmonization of our organs as much as possible in the given situation, and build our virtue account, waiting until internal/external energies that are more harmonious with our internal organs arrive to support what we want to accomplish. At times it may feel like all we are doing is filling the gaps, without any promise of progress. Be patient! It will happen when the gaps are filled. Compared to other options, it is a much easier, safer, faster, and wiser choice to fill our deficiencies and build our virtue account for when we need it.

How do I delete the old habits or information in my system?

Live by carrying out the right choices that we want to make, ones that are in line with the natural harmony of all living things. As we recognize and make the necessary changes, our information system files away the old information in its history section. It understands the new input as an improvement or adjustment, with the old information being no longer useful. If we continue with our new updated habits, the old information gets relegated to the history bin. For this part, we don't have to do anything more. It will slowly recede into a distant memory file.

However, before it fades away, our information system occasionally allows old habits to pop up and to get a final confirmation from us before fading away for good. Therefore, don't get confused by it. It just wants to make sure that we are happy with the changes we've made. We acknowledge this with a warm smile, and confirm it with, "I am good. You are free to go." With this confirmation we cut the tie, and allow it to move out of our current system and into a distant memory system. Now, it is done.

Chapter 6

How to Improve

How to Improve My Health

Whether we have a single dominant organ or a combination of strong organs, they are all based on our organs' internal body system. The external energies that come from our environment are not factored into this. (*See* "External Energies Entering Our Body," Chapter 7.)

Be aware that this isn't about right or wrong, or judging people's habits or their illnesses. We do this to understand and make improvements to our entire organ system, so we can finally blossom as individuals.

Each person will react differently to each food item, so be aware and take this into consideration when selecting food items.

When we decide to move forward with the food items that our organ system needs, our physical, mental, emotional, and spiritual well-being will improve.

What if I don't want to improve my health?

This may be the initial response from our dominating organ as we eat the foods that support our weaker organs. The dominant organ may fear the loss of control and power, so its habits will fight us every chance it gets as we move towards a more balanced and healthy body system. This is because the organ doesn't know any other way of existing.

Someone with a strong Stomach organ might say that they can eat anything and have no problems whatsoever. That may hold true for the Stomach. However, the weaker organs' deficiencies won't be taken into consideration due to monetary issues associated with the dominant Stomach.

Which Signals Should I Follow For Eating?

There are two kinds of craving signals.

One is an urgency coming from within us to let us know what we are lacking and what needs supplying. It is a very subtle signal, and the subtle message sometimes seems very illogical. The delivery is never sweet, never sugar coated, with no cunning, no explanation, or any justification for the craving. It is just a subtle message that arises from within. This is what we need to follow.

The other kind is an urgency that comes from the strong organs we carry, or the strong external energies influencing our five organs. These signals feel much more urgent, and it is designed to distract us from listening to the other more subtle message coming from within. Consequently, we supply the false signal instead because it feels very logical to answer the loudest craving. The other signal, if we notice it at all, doesn't make sense to us. This is why we are unable to balance our organ system to maintain better health.

Recognizing these two different signals can be tricky at times. Try both ways and learn to recognize the difference, and learn to follow the more subtle messages from within.

How do I know that I am eating the right foods for my body?

When we take in the foods that our organs need, we will know at some point to stop because we feel full and can't eat any more. Our body is giving us the signal to stop for now. We don't get to stuff more food in. Our body is saying, "That's enough, I am good." That's it. There are no confusing signals with this.

How do I know that I am consuming the wrong food items for my body?

When we supply the wrong food items to our body system, we can eat, eat, and eat and still feel unsatisfied. Something feels missing. No matter how much we eat, we are still looking for something to satisfy us. How many times have we searched for something to munch on (usually of unhealthy kind) after a meal?

The food that we just consumed sits in our stomach because none of the organs need it. And because it just sits there, we look for relief by eating something to move the old food out of our system. Unaware of what we are doing to ourselves, we repeat this cycle of eating the wrong foods in excess amounts over and over again. As for our organs, they don't see the need to absorb what doesn't benefit them.

This is the big difference between eating the foods that our body needs and what it doesn't need.

What's the result of taking the right foods for my body?

We will return to _____ as if we had always been healthy. And this may _____ mptoms we previously experienced. However, _____ g condition on a daily basis, we will recognize _____ le. It will be a smooth transition because it is a

_____ n?

_____ nd eat only the foods for our specific organs, _____ y faster afterward. This is the correct process. _____ izing the much needed food to convert it into

_____ us that it is still in need of that food. So, we _____ ng what has been used up.

_____ safe level and no longer in the deficit, it will _____ rmal portions.

_____ ive the sign to slow down, we are fully utilizing _____ improve the function of our entire body system.

How do I know for sure that my body is communicating with me?

As said earlier, when the food we eat is what our organ needs, we will know at some point when we shouldn't eat anymore. Our body is telling us that it's good for now. We don't get to stuff ourselves because the body firmly says, "No thanks. I am good."

How does my body communicate for the wrong foods?

So, we are eating the wrong foods, stuffing ourselves silly because we are not feeling satisfied for some reason no matter how much we eat. Something feels missing and we keep eating, hoping to fill the missing part. No such luck. Where is the signal?

Our weaker organs have been signaling the entire time. But we didn't get it. Why? Because our dominant organ intercepts the signal by sending out very loudly its own feelings and thoughts that have been translated as cravings. And by following these cravings sent by our dominant organ, we continue the whole entire cycle of eating excess foods that even the dominant organ doesn't need. These foods serve no other purpose than to be flushed down the toilet. We do this over and over again.

We don't have to *try* to be kind, pure, pretty, powerful, rich, or principled. And we don't need to ride the crazy roller-coaster that our thoughts and emotions take us on. The qualities we desire and the inner peace we need to function well will come naturally with a better organ system.

Just continue to take more of the beneficial food items until we reach the point of no discomfort. By then our body's signal system should be working better and much more efficiently.

***To expedite our health journey, let's create a virtue account by donating our time, talents and/or money to help people in need once our body system gets better. If we are already doing that, we increase the amount we give without thinking about having done it. Basically, don't let the left hand know what the right hand has done. The return on our investment will be greater than we might think.

If this is not possible, take five minutes from each day to reflect and be thankful, praying or sending out good will to all humanity. It will elevate us and all of humanity.

How to Improve My Health When Strong <u>Kidney-Kidney</u> Are Causing Problems

Follow these recommendations if you have strong Kidney organs already built in, and your life cycle is currently giving you an excess of this organ energy and causing health issues.

See Chapter 3, "Strong Kidney-Kidney," to see if you are experiencing the listed symptoms.

Step 1 Avoid all foods from the Kidney food list. This is a must.
Eat from the food lists of the following organs in the percentage indicated, per serving.

Stomach 40%
Heart 35%
Liver 10%
Lung 15%

Until your body system is brought into balance, your past habits will try to unbalance you on continual basis. Do not eat items that will cause imbalance in your body. For quite some time, you will have to fight to stay balanced but it will give you greater return on your health. However, this will be up to you. It's always your choice.

Step 2 Eat bitter and sweet tasting foods.
Maintain step one and add lamb into your daily diet.

Lamb Stew

Ingredients:
- 1 lb of lamb stew meat with fat trimmed off
- 3 small potatoes, diced
- 1 onion, diced
- 1 sweet yam, diced
- 1 medium carrot, diced
- 2 cups of cabbage, diced
- 2–3 cups of water
- salt or soup soy sauce (guk ganjang)
- crushed walnuts, pecans as garnish
- perilla seed powder if you can find it

Directions:
1. Boil the stew meat thoroughly and rinse the fat/grease off before transferring just the meat to a large pot or a slow cooker. (For slow cooker, dump everything in and cook for 6 hrs)
2. Add all the vegetables to the pot and pour in water
3. Bring to boil and then reduce heat and simmer for 1.5–2 hours.
4. Add salt and soy sauce to taste, 30 minutes before finishing.
5. Add a spoonful of crushed walnuts/pecans/perilla seed powder into the stew bowl and enjoy.

Lamb: At first, you may not like the smell of lamb, but it will get easier and you will find a way to remove the smell from the meat.

Please note: to reduce the risk of foodborne illness, it's important to cook the lamb meat thoroughly (well done) before consuming.

How often should I eat lamb?

1. Eat every day for 7 days.
2. Reduce to 3–4 times a week for 3–6 months, depending on the severity of the condition.
3. Then reduce to 2 times a week, or as needed.

Lamb with Sweet Fruit Sauce

Ingredients:
- package of lamb meat from Costco, around $20–$34, fat removed
- ginger, thumb-sized, peeled

Sauce ingredients:
- 1 cup of apricots fresh/dried
- 2 green apples
- 2 tbsp honey
- 1 tsp salt
- 1 cup dried cranberries
- 1 cup cabbage, diced

Directions:
1. Place defatted lamb meat into a large pot/pressure cooker with the ginger
2. Cook the meat thoroughly
3. Once finished cooking, remove from the pot and let it cool
4. cut into 1/2-inch slices

Sauce directions:
1. Put all the ingredients into a medium pot and bring to boil.
2. Reduce heat to medium low and cook for 30 min. to an hour. Make sure it doesn't boil over.
3. Once done, spoon over two slices of lamb and enjoy. You can also bake this in the oven for 30 min. at 350 degrees for more glazed lamb dish.
4. Eat with your choice of fresh vegetables and an optional 1–2 slices of bread.

Your body will take this food in and will be completely absorbed without any heartburn or indigestion. You will also get hungry very soon afterward. Why? Because your body needed it yesterday. For medicinal purpose, you only need two slices to work. If you eat more than that during a single meal, your body might waste the rest. Wait 2–3 hours before eating another serving. The body will take it in and use it.

Potato Pancake

Ingredients:
- 2–3 large potatoes
- 1/3 cup corn flour
- 1/3 cup tapioca flour
- 1/3 cup flour
- 1 tsp salt
- safflower oil
- water as needed

Directions:
1. Wash, peel, and grate the potatoes.
2. In a large bowl, combine all the ingredients.
3. Add enough water to make it a pancake batter consistency.
4. Ladle on to a well-greased pan and flip when golden brown.

How often should I eat this pancake?

Eat daily or as needed.

It will calm your body and you won't be as quick to anger. You will feel kinder, with more energy, clarity, and ability to see things in a brighter light. It's like finally reaching the shore after a long-distance swim.

As your eating habits change, you will notice that you eat fewer snacks because you feel generally satisfied. As a consequence, you may notice your grocery bill going down after several weeks.

After a few days or a few weeks, there should be noticeable improvement. Continue to take the beneficial foods until you reach a point of no discomfort.

You will return to better health conditions as if you had always been this healthy. And because a properly functioning body feels very natural and normal, and your body has nothing to complain about, you may not notice the changes as much. However, if you take note of your condition on a daily basis, you will recognize the improvements that you've already made.

***To expedite your health journey, create a virtue account by donating your time, talents, and/or money to help people in need once your body system gets better. If you are already doing that, increase the amount you do without thinking about having done it. Basically, don't let the left hand know what the right hand has done. The return on your investment will be greater than you might think.

If this is not possible, take five minutes from your day to reflect and be thankful, praying or sending out thoughts of good will to all humanity. It will elevate you and all of humanity.

How to Improve My Health When Strong
<u>Kidney-Heart</u> or <u>Heart-Kidney</u> Are Causing Problems

Follow these recommendations if you have strong Kidney and Heart organs already built in, and your life cycle is currently giving you an excess of these organ energies and causing health issues.

See Chapter 3, "Strong Kidney-Heart"/"Strong Heart-Kidney," to see if you are experiencing the listed symptoms.

Step 1 **Avoid all foods from the Kidney and Heart food lists.**

Eat from the food lists of the following organs in the percentage indicated, per serving.

Stomach 40%
Lung 45%
Liver 15%

Until your body system is brought into balance, your past habits will try to unbalance you on continual basis. Do not eat items that will cause imbalance in your body. For quite some time, you will have to fight to stay balanced, but it will give you greater return on your health. However, this will be up to you. It's always your choice.

Step 2 **Eat beef, fish, and a bit of sweet-tasting food.**

Eat these daily.
The results will be that you will feel stable and energized.

Special Hot Chicken Dish

Ingredients:
- 2 chicken breasts, thinly sliced
- 2 tbsp of chili powder/ Korean chili paste *go-chu-jang*
- 1 tsp salt
- black pepper to taste
- 1 large onion, sliced
- 1/2 cabbage, chopped/sliced
- 1 carrot, sliced

Directions:
1. Mix the chicken with the chili powder/paste, salt and pepper in a large frying pan and let it marinade as you prep other items.
2. Start cooking the contents of the frying pan on medium high, stirring.
3. Once the chicken in fully cooked, toss in the rest of the vegetables and stir fry for two minutes before turning off the heat.
4. Eat the chicken dish with brown rice or bread.

How often should I eat this chicken dish?

Eat as needed. At first, this dish may be too spicy for you and may take some getting used to.

After a few days or a few weeks, there should be noticeable improvement. Continue to take the beneficial foods until you reach a point of no discomfort.

You will return to better health conditions as if you had always been this healthy. And because a properly functioning body feels very natural and normal, and your body has nothing to complain about, you may not notice the changes as much. However, if you reflect or are aware of your condition on a daily basis, you will recognize the improvements that you've already made.

***To expedite your health journey, create a virtue account by donating your time, talents, and/or money to help people in need once your body system gets better. If you are already doing that, increase the amount you do without thinking about having done it. Basically, don't let the left hand know what the right hand has done. The return on your investment will be greater than you might think.

If this is not possible, take five minutes from your day to reflect and be thankful, praying or sending out thoughts of good will to all humanity. It will elevate you and all of humanity.

How to Improve My Health When Strong
<u>Kidney-Liver</u> or <u>Liver-Kidney</u> Are Causing Problems

Follow these recommendations if you have strong Kidney and Liver organs already built in, and your life cycle is currently giving you an excess of these organ energies and causing health issues.

See Chapter 3, "Strong Kidney-Liver"/"Strong Liver-Kidney," to see if you are experiencing the listed symptoms.

Step 1 **Avoid all foods from the Kidney and Liver food lists. This is a must. Eat from the food lists of the following organs in the percentage indicated, per serving.**

Stomach 40%
Lung 30%
Heart 30%

Until your body system is brought into balance, your past habits will try to unbalance you on continual basis. Do not eat items that will cause imbalance in your body. For quite some time, you will have to fight to stay balanced, but it will give you greater return on your health. However, this will be up to you. It's always your choice.

Step 2 **Eat bitter and sweet-tasting foods.**
Maintain step one and add lamb into your daily diet. Some may have to continue this until all the previous symptoms are gone. After that, reduce the lamb to 3 times a week.
**Use 1 tbsp of Chinese black bean paste by Chung Jung Won for stir-fried vegetables or stew. Eat daily to improve the body and make it warmer.

Lamb Beef Stew

Ingredients:
- 1 lb. of lamb stew meat with fat trimmed off
- 1/2 lb. of beef stew meat, fat trimmed off
- 3 small potatoes, diced
- 1 onion, diced
- 1 sweet yam, diced
- 1 medium carrot, diced
- 2 cups of cabbage, diced
- 2–3 cups of water
- salt or soup soy sauce (guk ganjang)
- chili pepper

Directions:
1. Slightly boil the stew meat and rinse the fat/grease off before transferring just the meat to a large pot or a slow cooker. (For slow cooker, dump everything in and cook for 6 hrs)
2. Add beef and all the vegetables to the pot and pour in water.
3. Bring to boil and then reduce heat and simmer for 1.5–2 hours.
4. Add salt and soy sauce to taste, 30 minutes before finishing.
5. Add chili pepper

(Strong Kidney-Liver or Liver-Kidney, continued)

At first, you may not like the smell of lamb, but it will get easier and you will find a way to remove the smell from the meat.

Please note: to reduce the risk of foodborne illness, it's important to cook the lamb meat thoroughly (well done) before consuming.

How often should I eat this stew?

Eat this daily. In a few days to a week, your intensity will mellow out, and you will become less impatient, and more able to find room to listen to others as you continue.

When you reach that stage, reduce to twice a week.

Until your body system is brought into balance, your past habits will try to unbalance you on continual basis. Do not eat items that will cause imbalance in your body. For quite some time, you will have to fight to stay balanced, but it will give you greater return on your health. However, this will be up to you. It's always your choice.

As your eating habits change, you will notice that you eat less of other things such as snacks because you feel generally satisfied. As a consequence, you may notice your grocery bill going down after several weeks.

After a few days or a few weeks, there should be noticeable improvement. Continue to take the beneficial foods until you reach a point of no discomfort.

You will return to better health conditions as if you had always been this healthy. And because a properly functioning body feels very natural and normal, and your body has nothing to complain about, you may not notice the changes as much. However, if you take note of your condition on a daily basis, you will recognize the improvements that you've already made.

***To expedite your health journey, create a virtue account by donating your time, talents, and/or money to help people in need once your body system gets better. If you are already doing them, increase the amount you do without thinking about having done it. Basically, don't let the left hand know what the right hand has done. The return on your investment will be greater than you might think.

If this is not possible, take five minutes from your day to reflect and be thankful, praying or sending out thoughts of good will to all humanity. It will elevate you and all of humanity.

How to Improve My Health When Strong
<u>Kidney-Lung</u> or <u>Lung-Kidney</u> Are Causing Problems

Follow these recommendations if you have strong Kidney and Lung organs already built in, and your life cycle is currently giving you an excess of these organ energies and causing health issues.

See Chapter 3, "Strong Kidney-Lung"/"Strong Lung-Kidney" to see if you are experiencing the listed symptoms.

Step 1 Avoid all foods from the Kidney and Lung food lists.

Avoid wifi routers and living near substations and cell towers.

Eat from the food lists of the following organs in the percentage indicated, per serving.

Stomach 30%
Heart 40%
Liver 30%

Step 2 Eat the following special dish for this body type.

Lamb with Sweet Fruit Sauce

Ingredients:
- package of lamb meat from Costco, around $20–$34, fat removed
- ginger, thumb-sized, peeled

Sauce ingredients:
- 1 cup of apricots fresh/dried
- 2 green apples
- 2 tbsp honey
- 1 tsp salt
- 1 cup dried cranberries
- 1 cup cabbage, diced

__Please note__: to reduce the risk of foodborne illness, it's important to cook the lamb meat thoroughly (well done) before consuming.

Directions:
1. Place defatted lamb meat into a large pot/pressure cooker with the ginger.
2. Cook the meat all the way.
3. Once finished cooking, remove from the pot and let it cool.
4. Cut into 1/2-inch slices.

Sauce Directions:
1. Put all the ingredients into a medium pot and bring to boil.
2. Reduce heat to medium low and cook for 30 min. to an hour. Make sure it doesn't boil over.
3. Once done, spoon over two slices of lamb and enjoy. You can also bake this in the oven for 30 min. at 350 degrees for a more glazed lamb dish.
4. Eat with your choice of fresh vegetables and an optional 1–2 slices of bread.

How often should I eat the lamb?

Eat 2–3 times a week.

(Strong Kidney-Lung or Lung-Kidney, continued)

Your body will take this food in and will be completely absorbed without any heartburn or indigestion. You will also get hungry very soon afterward. Why? Because your body needed it yesterday. For medicinal purpose, you only need two slices to work. If you eat more than that during a single meal, your body might waste the rest. Wait 2–3 hours before eating another serving, if you must, but be sure to not go overboard. The body will take it in and use it.

Until your body system is brought into balance, your past habits will try to unbalance you on continual basis. Do not eat items that will cause imbalance in your body. For quite some time, you will have to fight to stay balanced, but it will give you greater return on your health. However, this will be up to you. It's always your choice.

As your eating habits change, you will notice that you eat less of other things such as snacks because you feel generally satisfied. As a consequence, you may notice your grocery bill going down after several weeks.

Tips on Mung Bean and Millet Pancakes

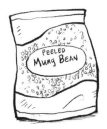 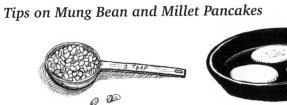

You can find peeled split mung beans online or in Asian grocery stores.

They are tiny and yellow in color.

The batter should be similar to regular pancake batter. Make sure the pan is hot and there's enough oil when you start.

Mung Bean and Millet Pancake

Ingredients:
- 2 cups peeled mung beans
- 1/2 cup of millet
- 2 medium potatoes
- 1/2 cup of tapioca flour
- 1 egg
- 1/4 cup cranberries
- good quality salt
- olive and sunflower seed oil

Directions:
1. Rinse and soak the peeled mung beans and the millet in 2–3 cups of warm water for 4 hours.
2. Add into the blender/food processor, the soaked mung beans, millet, potatoes, tapioca flour, egg, salt, cranberries, and enough water to just cover the ingredients. Blend to fine consistency.
3. Pour several tbsp of oil on to a hot pan, and ladle in the bean mixture to make small- to medium-sized pancakes. Flip once the edges turn golden brown.
4. If the bean batter is too watery, you can add flour for better consistency. If you add other items, it will change the medicinal property of this dish.
5. Huckleberries are a good match to eat with this pancake for this body type.

(Strong Kidney-Lung or Lung-Kidney, continued)

How often should I eat this pancake?

Daily.

It will calm your body and you won't be as quick to anger. You will feel kinder, with more energy, clarity, and improved muscle and joint powers.

After a few days or a few weeks, there should be noticeable improvement. Continue to take the beneficial foods until you reach a point of no discomfort.

You will return to better health conditions as if you had always been this healthy. And because a properly functioning body feels very natural and normal, and your body has nothing to complain about, you may not notice the changes as much. However, if you take note of your condition on a daily basis, you will recognize the improvements that you've already made.

***To expedite your health journey, create a virtue account by donating your time, talents, and/or money to help people in need once your body system gets better. If you are already doing that, increase the amount you do without thinking about having done it. Basically, don't let the left hand know what the right hand has done. The return on your investment will be greater than you might think.

If this is not possible, take five minutes from your day to reflect and be thankful, praying or sending out thoughts of good will to all humanity. It will elevate you and all of humanity.

How to Improve My Health When Strong
<u>Kidney-Stomach</u> or <u>Stomach-Kidney</u> Are Causing Problems

Follow these recommendations if you have strong Kidney and Stomach organs already built in, and your life cycle is currently giving you an excess of these organ energies and causing health issues.

See Chapter 3, "Strong Kidney-Stomach"/"Strong Stomach-Kidney," to see if you are experiencing the listed symptoms.

Step 1 **Avoid all foods from the Kidney and Stomach food lists.**

Eat from the food lists of the following organs in the percentage indicated, per serving.

Heart 40%
Liver 30%
Lung 30%

Until your body system is brought into balance, your past habits will try to unbalance you on continual basis. Do not eat items that will cause imbalance in your body. For quite some time, you will have to fight to stay balanced, but it will give you greater return on your health. However, this will be up to you. It's always your choice.

Step 2 **Eat bitter and sweet-tasting foods.**
Maintain step one and add lamb into your diet 2–3 times a week. Some may have to continue this until all the previous symptoms are gone.

Lamb Stew

Ingredients:
- 1 lb. of lamb stew meat with fat trimmed off
- 3 small potatoes, diced
- 1 onion, diced
- 1 sweet yam, diced
- 1 medium carrot, diced
- 2 cups of cabbage, diced
- 2–3 cups of water
- salt or soup soy sauce (guk ganjang)
- crushed walnuts, pecans as garnish
- perilla seed powder if you can find it

Directions:
1. Slightly boil the stew meat and rinse the fat/grease off before transferring just the meat to a large pot or a slow cooker. (For slow cooker, dump everything in and cook for 6 hrs)
2. Add all the vegetables to the pot and pour in water.
3. Bring to boil and then reduce heat and simmer for 1.5–2 hours.
4. Add salt and soy sauce to taste, 30 minutes before finishing.
5. Add a spoonful of crushed walnuts/pecans/perilla seed powder into the stew bowl and enjoy.

(Strong Kidney-Stomach or Stomach-Kidney, continued)

At first, you may not like the smell of lamb, but it will get easier and you will find a way to remove the smell from the meat.

Please note: to reduce the risk of foodborne illness, it's important to cook the lamb meat thoroughly (well done) before consuming.

How often should I eat this stew?

Eat this 2–3 times a week. Your intensity will mellow out, and you'll become less impatient and able to find more room to listen to others as you continue.

**Use 1 tbsp of Chinese black bean paste by Chung Jung Won for stir fried vegetables or stew.

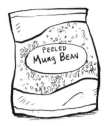

Tips on Mung Bean and Millet Pancakes

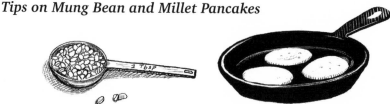

You can find peeled split mung beans online or in Asian grocery stores.

They are tiny and yellow in color.

The batter should be similar to regular pancake batter. Make sure the pan is hot and there's enough oil when you start.

Mung Bean and Millet Pancake

Ingredients:
- 2 cups peeled mung beans
- 1/2 cup of Indian millet
- 2 medium potatoes
- 1/2 cup corn flour
- 1 egg
- good quality salt
- olive and sunflower seed oil

Directions:
1. Rinse and soak the peeled mung beans and the millet in 2–3 cups of warm water for 4 hours.
2. Add into the blender/food processor, the soaked mung beans, millet, potatoes, egg, corn flour, salt, and enough water to just cover the ingredients. Blend to fine consistency.
3. Pour several tbsp of oil on to a hot pan, and ladle in the bean mixture into whatever size pancake you want. Flip once the edges turn golden brown.
4. If the bean batter is too watery, you can add flour for better consistency. If you add other items, it will change the medicinal property of this dish.
5. Apricots and plums are a good combination to eat with this pancake for this body type.

How often should I eat this pancake?

As needed.

It will calm your body and you won't be as quick to anger. You will feel kinder, with more energy, clarity, and ability to see things in a brighter light. It's like you're finally reaching the shore after a long-distance swim.

As your eating habits change, you will notice that you eat less of other things such as snacks because you feel generally satisfied. As a consequence, you may notice your grocery bill going down after several weeks.

After a few days or a few weeks, there should be noticeable improvement. Continue to take the beneficial foods until you reach a point of no discomfort.

You will return to better health conditions as if you had always been this healthy. And because a properly functioning body feels very natural and normal, and your body has nothing to complain about, you may not notice the changes as much. However, if you take note of your condition on a daily basis, you will recognize the improvements that you've already made.

***To expedite your health journey, create a virtue account by donating your time, talents, and/or money to help people in need once your body system gets better. If you are already doing that, increase the amount you do without thinking about having done it. Basically, don't let the left hand know what the right hand has done. The return on your investment will be greater than you might think.

If this is not possible, take five minutes from your day to reflect and be thankful, praying or sending out thoughts of good will to all humanity. It will elevate you and all of humanity.

How to Improve My Health When Strong <u>Heart-Heart</u> Are Causing Problems

Follow these recommendations if you have a strong Heart organ already built in, and your life cycle is currently giving you an excess of this organ energy and causing health issues.

See Chapter 3, "Strong Heart-Heart" to see if you are experiencing the listed symptoms.

Step 1 Avoid all foods from the Heart food list. This is a must.

Eat from the food lists of the following organs in the percentage indicated, per serving.

Kidney 30%
Liver 30%
Lung 40%

Step 2 Drink aloe vera juice and berry juice (no sugar added)
Start with 3 x 8oz glass
Some situations require 5 glasses to maintain the balance

Until your body system is brought into balance, your past habits will try to unbalance you on continual basis. Do not eat items that will cause imbalance in your body. For quite some time, you will have to fight to stay balanced, but it will give you greater return on your health. However, this will be up to you. It's always your choice.

Seaweed and Scallop Soup

Ingredients:
- 1/2 cup dried seaweed, cut into 2" lengths
- 1/2 cup dried mushrooms
- 1 can of clams/clam juice
- 5 scallops
- 1/2 cup of radish, thinly sliced
- 1/4 cup dried cranberries
- good quality salt/soup soy sauce (guk-ganjang)
- mung bean sprouts (optional)
- 1 tbsp crushed pine nuts/almonds (optional)

Directions:
1. Soak the dried seaweed in warm water for 10 min. Rinse and put into a large pot with 7 cups of water and bring to boil.
2. Add mushrooms, clams/clam juice, scallops, radishes, and cranberries.
3. Season with salt/soup soy sauce and let it cook for additional 15 min.
4. Add mung bean sprouts 2 min. prior to serving (optional).
5. Add a spoonful of crushed pine nuts/almonds to the bowl before eating (optional).

How often should I eat this seaweed scallop soup dish?

Eat daily.

*Seaweed and cucumber salad is also highly recommended.

Adzuki Bean Juice

Ingredients:

- 2 cups of adzuki beans, rinsed well
- large cloth/muslin bag
- 5 cups of water
- 2 tsp salt

Directions:

1. Put the rinsed adzuki beans into the muslin/cotton bag.
2. Put the bag of beans into a large pot or pressure cooker.
3. Add water and salt, and bring to boil on high with lid closed.
4. Once it boils, bring the heat to medium-low and cook for an hour.
5. Refrigerate after cooling to room temperature and transferring the liquid to a storage container.
6. You can reuse the remaining beans by simply cooking it again with 4 cups of water and salt, using same procedure.
7. Then discard the beans.

How often should I drink this?

Religiously drink 8 oz daily.

After a few days or a few weeks, there should be noticeable improvement. Continue to take the beneficial foods until you reach a point of no discomfort.

You will return to better health conditions as if you had always been this healthy. And because a properly functioning body feels very natural and normal, and your body has nothing to complain about, you may not notice the changes as much. However, if you reflect or are aware of your condition on a daily basis, you will recognize the improvements that you've already made.

Note: After you eat the special dishes and do the daily intake of your organ foods, you will find that you get hungry faster than before. This is the correct process. Because your body is being fully utilized by the organs, they are simply letting you know that they are ready for more. Keep eating until your body tells you to stop, that it has enough for now. Instead of being wasted, all the food you have eaten is being fully used to provide you with better functioning body system.

***To expedite your health journey, create a virtue account by donating your time, talents, and/or money to help people in need once your body system gets better. If you are already doing them, increase the amount you do without thinking about having done it. Basically, don't let the left hand know what the right hand has done. The return on your investment will be greater than you might think.

If this is not possible, take five minutes from your day to reflect and be thankful, praying or sending out thoughts of good will to all humanity. It will elevate you and all of humanity.

How to Improve My Health When Strong
<u>Heart-Liver</u> or <u>Liver-Heart</u> Are Causing Problems

Follow these recommendations if you have strong Heart and Liver organs already built in, and your life cycle is currently giving you an excess of these organ energies and causing health issues.

See Chapter 3, "Strong Heart-Liver"/"Strong Liver-Heart," to see if you are experiencing the listed symptoms.

Step 1 **Avoid all foods from the Heart and Liver food lists. This is a must.**

> **Eat from the food lists of the following organs in the percentage indicated, per serving.**
>
> **Kidney 30%**
> **Stomach 30%**
> **Lung 40%**

Step 2 **Drink aloe vera juice and berry juice (no sugar added)**
Start with 3 x 8oz glass
Some situations require more than 3 glasses to maintain the balance

> Until your body system is brought into balance, your past habits will try to unbalance you on continual basis. Do not eat items that will cause imbalance in your body. For quite some time, you will have to fight to stay balanced, but it will give you greater return on your health. However, this will be up to you. It's always your choice.

Following is a special soup for this body type. It is an inexpensive way to cool down, circulate, and soothe the system. This soup will make you feel comfortable both emotionally and physically.

Seaweed and Abalone Soup

Ingredients:
- 1/2 cup dried seaweed, cut into 2" lengths
- 1/2 cup dried mushroom
- 1 can of clams/clam juice
- 1/4 to 1/2 cup abalone, chopped
- 1/2 cup of radish, thinly sliced
- 1/4 cup dried cranberry
- good quality salt/soup soy sauce (guk-ganjang)
- mung bean sprouts (optional)
- 1 tbsp crushed pine nuts/almonds (optional)

Directions:
1. Soak the dried seaweed in warm water for 10 min. Rinse and put into a large pot with 5 cups of water and bring to boil.
2. Add mushrooms, clams/clam juice, abalone, radishes, and cranberries.
3. Season with salt/soup soy sauce and let it cook for additional 15 min.
4. Add mung bean sprouts 2 min. prior to serving (optional).
5. Add a spoonful of crushed pine nuts/almonds to the bowl before eating (optional).

How often should I eat this Seaweed and Abalone Soup dish?

Eat daily.

*Seaweed and cucumber salad is also highly recommended.

After a few days or a few weeks, there should be noticeable improvement. Continue to take the beneficial foods until you reach a point of no discomfort.

You will return to better health conditions as if you had always been this healthy. And because a properly functioning body feels very natural and normal, and your body has nothing to complain about, you may not notice the changes as much. However, if you take note of your condition on a daily basis, you will recognize the improvements that you've already made.

Note: After you eat the special dishes and do the daily intake of your organ foods, you will find that you get hungry faster than before. This is the correct process. Because your body is being fully utilized by the organs, they are simply letting you know that they are ready for more. Keep eating until your body tells you to stop, that it has enough for now. Instead of being wasted, all the food you have eaten is being fully used to provide you with better functioning body system.

A word of caution: until the body is convinced of continual supply, it may not take it in right away. So, you may feel full for a bit until the body absorbs the food.

***To expedite your health journey, create a virtue account by donating your time, talents, and/or money to help people in need once your body system gets better. If you are already doing that, increase the amount you do without thinking about having done it. Basically, don't let the left hand know what the right hand has done. The return on your investment will be greater than you might think.

If this is not possible, take five minutes from your day to reflect and be thankful, praying or sending out thoughts of good will to all humanity. It will elevate you and all of humanity.

How to Improve My Health When Strong
<u>Heart-Lung</u> or <u>Lung-Heart</u> Are Causing Problems

Follow these recommendations if you have strong Heart and Lung organs already built in, and your life cycle is currently giving you an excess of these organ energies and causing health issues.

See Chapter 3, "Strong Heart-Lung"/"Strong Lung-Heart" to see if you are experiencing the listed symptoms.

Step 1 Avoid all foods from the Heart and Lung food lists. This is a must.

Avoid wifi routers and living near substations and cell towers.

Eat from the food lists of the following organs in the percentage indicated, per serving.

Stomach 30%
Kidney 30%
Liver 40%

Until your body system is brought into balance, your past habits will try to unbalance you on a continual basis. Do not eat items that will cause imbalance in your body. For quite some time, you will have to fight to stay balanced, but it will give you greater return on your health. However, this will be up to you. It's always your choice.

Step 2 *If possible, Susin Ogapy Royal is highly recommended, but it is only available through <u>Susinogapy</u> in South Korea, the only company that makes them this high quality that I've come across. It provides safe recovery of the liver, immune, and Kidney systems, without any side effects. I've experienced this product myself and through others for over 20 years. I have no personal connection with this company. It is just that there are no other company that offers this product at this exceptional level of quality. This is the only thing they sell and have spent their lifetime perfecting it. It is certainly not inexpensive. However, when one considers the quality of this herb product, it is a bargain.

Chicken, Clam, and Cabbage Soup

Ingredients:
- 2 chicken breasts, diced/sliced.
- 1 can of clams/clam juice
- 3 kombu/seaweed pieces 2"x2"
- 1/2 cabbage, chopped
- 1/2 cup dried mushrooms
- 2 tsp salt/2 tbsp soup soy sauce
- 2 eggs
- 5 cups water

Directions:
1. Trim the fat off the chicken breast.
2. On a hot pan, lightly sear the chicken breasts on both sides.
3. Dice or slice the chicken breasts to bite-sized pieces.
4. In a large pot, combine chicken, clams, cabbage, dried mushrooms, seaweed, salt/soup soy sauce, and water, cooking for 20–30 minutes.
5. Add beaten eggs to the soup right before turning off the stove.

How often should I eat this?

Eat daily.

You will be kinder, calmer, more alive, energized, and with greater clarity and improved memory and Kidney systems.

After a few days or a few weeks, there should be noticeable improvement. Continue to take the beneficial foods until you reach a point of no discomfort.

You will return to better health conditions as if you had always been this healthy. And because a properly functioning body feels very natural and normal, and your body has nothing to complain about, you may not notice the changes as much. However, if you take note of your condition on a daily basis, you will recognize the improvements that you've already made.

***To expedite your health journey, create a virtue account by donating your time, talents, and/or money to help people in need once your body system gets better. If you are already doing that, increase the amount you do without thinking about having done it. Basically, don't let the left hand know what the right hand has done. The return on your investment will be greater than you might think.

If this is not possible, take five minutes from your day to reflect and be thankful, praying or sending out thoughts of good will to all humanity. It will elevate you and all of humanity.

How to Improve My Health When Strong
Heart-Stomach or Stomach-Heart Are Causing Problems

Follow these recommendations if you have strong Heart and Stomach organs already built in, and your life cycle is currently giving you an excess of these organ energies and causing health issues.

See Chapter 3, "Strong Heart-Stomach"/"Strong Stomach-Heart," to see if you are experiencing the listed symptoms.

Step 1 **Avoid all foods from the Heart and Stomach food lists. This is a must.**

> **Eat from the food lists of the following organs in the percentage indicated, per serving.**
>
> **Kidney 35%**
> **Liver 35%**
> **Lung 30%**
>
> Until your body system is brought into balance, your past habits will try to unbalance you on a continual basis. Do not eat items that will cause imbalance in your body. For quite some time, you will have to fight to stay balanced, but it will give you greater return on your health. However, this will be up to you. It's always your choice.

Step 2 **This is an inexpensive way to cool down the inner temperature and soothe the system. This soup will instantly make you feel more comfortable both physically and emotionally.**

Seaweed and Scallop Soup

Ingredients:
- 1/2 cup dried seaweed, cut into 2" lengths
- 1/2 cup dried mushrooms
- 1 can of clams/clam juice
- 2–3 scallops
- 2 cups of radish, thinly sliced
- 1 tsp sesame seed oil
- good quality salt/soup soy sauce (guk-ganjang)
- mung bean sprouts (optional)
- 1/4 cup crushed pine nuts/almonds (optional)

Directions:
1. Soak the dried seaweed in warm water for 10 min. Rinse and put into a large pot with 7 cups of water and bring to boil.
2. Add mushrooms, clams/clam juice, sesame oil, walnuts, scallops, and radishes.
3. Season with salt/soup soy sauce and let it cook for additional 15 min.
4. Add mung bean sprouts 2 min. prior to serving (optional).
5. Add a spoonful of crushed pine nuts/almonds to the bowl before eating (optional).

Another Recommended Seaweed Soup

Ingredients:

- 1/2 cup of dried seaweed cut into 2" lengths
- 1/4 cup of dried cranberries
- 1/4 cup dried anchovies
- 1/2 cup of dried mushrooms
- high quality salt/soy sauce

Directions:

1. Soak the dried seaweed in warm water for 10 min. Rinse and put into a large pot with 7 cups of water and bring to boil.
2. Add cranberries, anchovies, and dried mushrooms.
3. Season with salt/soup soy sauce and let it cook for additional 15 min.

---

*Eating seaweed and cucumber salad also highly recommended.

How often should I eat this soup?

Eat daily.

Adzuki Bean Juice

Ingredients:

- 2 cups of adzuki* beans, rinsed well
- large cloth/muslin bag
- 5 cups of water
- 2 tsp salt

Directions:

1. Put the rinsed adzuki beans into the muslin/cotton bag.
2. Put the bag of beans into a large pot or pressure cooker.
3. Add water and salt, and bring to boil on high with the lid closed.
4. Once it boils, bring the heat to medium-low and cook for an hour.
5. Cool to room temperature before transferring the liquid to a storage container.
6. Refrigerate.
7. You can reuse the remaining beans by simply cooking it again with 4 cups of water and salt, using same procedure.
8. Then discard the beans.

*Adzuki beans are small red beans originating from Asia, and should not be confused with kidney beans which are larger and kidney shaped.

How often should I drink this?

Religiously drink 8 oz daily.

If you find it difficult to follow this diet, try sharing something with others through good deeds. It will create room inside so you can grow. A good deed will definitely help you head in the right direction.

A person with this body system is sunshine to many, especially those looking for warmth. Take care of yourself first!

After a few days or a few weeks, there should be noticeable improvement. Continue to take the beneficial foods until you reach a point of no discomfort.

You will return to better health conditions as if you had always been this healthy. And because a properly functioning body feels very natural and normal, and your body has nothing to complain about, you may not notice the changes as much. However, if you reflect or are aware of your condition on a daily basis, you will recognize the improvements that you've already made.

***To expedite your health journey, create a virtue account by donating your time, talents, and/or money to help people in need once your body system gets better. If you are already doing that, increase the amount you do without thinking about having done it. Basically, don't let the left hand know what the right hand has done. The return on your investment will be greater than you might think.

If this is not possible, take five minutes from your day to reflect and be thankful, praying or sending out thoughts of good will to all humanity. It will elevate you and all of humanity.

How to Improve My Health When Strong Liver-Liver Are Causing Problems

Follow these recommendations if you have a strong Liver organ already built in, and your life cycle is currently giving you an excess of this organ energy and causing health issues.

See Chapter 3, "Strong Liver-Liver" to see if you are experiencing the listed symptoms.

Step 1 Avoid all foods from the Liver food list if you want better health. The strong stubbornness of the Liver energy will challenge the food list, bringing in all the logic at its disposal to undermine and question it. Be aware.

Eat from the food lists of the following organs in the percentage indicated per serving.

Stomach 30%
Lung 30%
Heart 25%
Kidney 15%

Until your body system is brought into balance, your past habits will try to unbalance you on continual basis. Do not eat items that will cause imbalance in your body. For quite some time, you will have to fight to stay balanced, but it will give you greater return on your health. However, this will be up to you. It's always your choice.

Step 2 Eating sweet, bitter, and clear tasting foods is beneficial.

1. Make sure to follow Step 1 above.
2. Propolis paste 2–3 times a day.
3. Gingko powder 1 tbsp 3 times a day. (Let it steep in warm to hot water, or mix with other drinks like coffee, hot cocoa, green tea, and ginger tea with honey. The powder is sort of bitter by itself, but someone with this Liver body type can take it with something sweet and have the body utilize it fully.)
4. Or, drink ginseng with aloe vera juice (no sugar added).
5. Add extra hot spicy seasoning into your daily diet.

How often should I do this?

Daily and religiously.

(Strong Liver-Liver, continued)

You will find your logic and its accompanying knowledge fight every moment of this diet. However, as you find yourself getting healthier, your logic will be left confused and puzzled by the change.

The result will be that as you progress, your physical presentation, emotional display, and mental thought process will improve. You will become less one-sided and will develop broader perspective.

After a few days or a few weeks, there should be noticeable improvement. Continue to take the beneficial foods until you reach a point of no discomfort.

You will return to better health conditions as if you had always been this healthy. And because a properly functioning body feels very natural and normal, and your body has nothing to complain about, you may not notice the changes as much. However, if you take note of your condition on a daily basis, you will recognize the improvements that you've already made.

***To expedite your health journey, create a virtue account by donating your time, talents, and/or money to help people in need once your body system gets better. If you are already doing that, increase the amount you do without thinking about having done it. Basically, don't let the left hand know what the right hand has done. The return on your investment will be greater than you might think.

If this is not possible, take five minutes from your day to reflect and be thankful, praying or sending out thoughts of good will to all humanity. It will elevate you and all of humanity.

How to Improve My Health When Strong
<u>Liver-Lung</u> or <u>Lung-Liver</u> Are Causing Problems

Follow these recommendations if you have strong Liver and Lung organs already built in, and your life cycle is currently giving you an excess of these organ energies and causing health issues.

See Chapter 3, "Strong Liver-Lung"/"Strong Lung-Liver," to see if you are experiencing the listed symptoms.

Step 1   Avoid all foods from the Liver and Lung food lists if you want better health.

Eat from the food lists of the following organs in the percentage indicated, per serving.

Stomach 40%
Heart 40%
Kidney 20%

Until your body system is brought into balance, your past habits will try to unbalance you on continual basis. Do not eat items that will cause imbalance in your body. For quite some time, you will have to fight to stay balanced, but it will give you greater return on your health. However, this will be up to you. It's always your choice.

Step 2   **Eat sweet and bitter tasting foods.**
1. **Make sure to follow Step 1 above**
2. **Propolis paste 2–3 times a day**
3. **Coffee, hot cocoa, green tea, grapes, grapefruit**
4. **Ginseng**

Lamb and Cabbage Soup

Ingredients:
- 2 lamb steaks
- 1 full head of cabbage, sliced/chopped
- 2 carrots, chopped
- 1 onion, chopped
- 1 large potato, diced
- 1/2 cup of dried mushrooms
- 4–5 slices of ginger
- good quality salt
- 1/2 cup of crushed cashew nuts

Directions:
1. Boil the lamb meat in water. After it's cooked all the way, rinse under running water. Throw away the broth and fat.
2. Slice the meat into bite sized pieces and put into a large pot or crock pot.
3. Add cabbage, carrots, onion, potato, dried mushrooms, ginger, salt, and cashews to the pot and bring to a boil.
4. Turn down the heat to medium-low and simmer for 30–40 minutes. Serve in a bowl and enjoy.

***Please note**: to reduce the risk of foodborne illness, it's important to cook the lamb meat thoroughly (well done) before consuming.*

This soup will satisfy your body's needs as it utilizes everything in it. However, you will get hungry quickly because your body needs a lot more of the soup. You can eat as much as you need until you reach the point where your body tells you "enough." At that point the hunger will slow down and your body will begin to circulate rapidly. Are you ready for that?

How often should I eat the soup?

Eat 2–3 times a week.

The body will return to its original warmth and will circulate.

The result will be that as you progress, your physical presentation, emotional display, and mental thought process will improve. You will become less one-sided and will develop broader perspective.

After a few days or a few weeks, there should be noticeable improvement. Continue to take the beneficial foods until you reach a point of no discomfort.

You will return to better health conditions as if you had always been this healthy. And because a properly functioning body feels very natural and normal, and your body has nothing to complain about, you may not notice the changes as much. However, if you take note of your condition on a daily basis, you will recognize the improvements that you've already made.

***To expedite your health journey, create a virtue account by donating your time, talents, and/or money to help people in need once your body system gets better. If you are already doing that, increase the amount you do without thinking about having done it. Basically, don't let the left hand know what the right hand has done. The return on your investment will be greater than you might think.

If this is not possible, take five minutes from your day to reflect and be thankful, praying or sending out thoughts of good will to all humanity. It will elevate you and all of humanity.

How to Improve My Health When Strong
<u>Liver-Stomach</u> or <u>Stomach-Liver</u> Are Causing Problems

Follow these recommendations if you have strong Liver and Stomach organs already built in, and your life cycle is currently giving you an excess of this organ energy and causing health issues.

See Chapter 3, "Strong Liver-Stomach"/"Strong Stomach-Liver," to see if you are experiencing the listed symptoms.

Step 1 Avoid all foods from the Liver and Stomach food lists if you want better health.

Eat from the food lists of the following organs in the percentage indicated, per serving.

Lung 30%
Heart 30%
Kidney 40%

Until your body system is brought into balance, your past habits will try to unbalance you on continual basis. Do not eat items that will cause imbalance in your body. For quite some time, you will have to fight to stay balanced, but it will give you greater return on your health. However, this will be up to you. It's always your choice.

Step 2 Eating bitter, cool, and clear tasting foods are beneficial.

1. Gingko powder 1 tbsp a day. (Let it steep in warm to hot water, or mix with other drinks like coffee, hot coco, green tea, and ginger tea sweetened lightly with honey. The powder is sort of bitter to drink by itself.)
2. Or, drink ginseng with aloe vera juice (no sugar added)
3. Add extra hot spicy seasoning into your daily diet.

Adzuki Bean Juice

Ingredients:

- 2 cups of adzuki beans, rinsed well
- large cloth/muslin bag
- 5 cups of water
- 2 tsp salt

Directions:

1. Put the rinsed adzuki beans into the muslin/cotton bag.
2. Put the bag of beans into a large pot or pressure cooker.
3. Add water and salt, and bring to boil on high with lid closed.
4. Once it boils, bring the heat to medium-low and cook for an hour.
5. Refrigerate after cooling to room temperature and transferring the liquid to a storage container.
6. You can reuse the remaining beans by simply cooking it again with 4 cups of water and salt, using same procedure.
7. Then discard the beans.

(Strong Liver-Stomach or Stomach-Liver, continued)

How often should I drink this?

Drink 4–8 oz daily and religiously.

Seaweed and Bone Marrow Soup

Ingredients:
- 1/2 cup dried seaweed, cut into 2" lengths
- 1/2 cup of dried mushrooms
- 1/2 cup of scallops
- 1 can of clams/clam juice
- 2 cups of radish, thinly sliced
- 1 cup beef bone broth
- 1 tsp sesame seed oil
- good quality salt/soup soy sauce (guk-ganjang)
- mung bean sprouts (optional)
- 1/4 cup crushed pine nuts/almonds (optional)

Directions:
1. Soak the dried seaweed in warm water for 10 min. Rinse and put into a large pot with 7 cups of water and bring to boil.
2. Add mushrooms, clams/clam juice, sesame oil, scallops, and radishes.
3. Season with salt/soup soy sauce and let it cook for additional 15 min.
4. Add mung bean sprouts 2 min. prior to serving (optional).
5. Add a spoonful of crushed pine nuts/almonds to the bowl before eating (optional).

How often should I eat this Seaweed and Bone Marrow Soup dish?

Eat daily.

*Seaweed and cucumber salad is also highly recommended.

You will find that your logic and its accompanying knowledge fight every moment of this diet. However, as you find yourself getting healthier, your logic will be left confused and puzzled by the change.

The result will be that as you progress, your physical presentation, emotional display, and mental thought process will improve. You will become less one-sided and will develop broader perspective.

After a few days or a few weeks, there should be noticeable improvement. Continue to take the beneficial foods until you reach a point of no discomfort.

***To expedite your health journey, create a virtue account by donating your time, talents, and/or money to help people in need once your body system gets better. If you are already doing that, increase the amount you do without thinking about having done it. Basically, don't let the left hand know what the right hand has done. The return on your investment will be greater than you might think.

If this is not possible, take five minutes from your day to reflect and be thankful, praying or sending out thoughts of good will to all humanity. It will elevate you and all of humanity.

How to Improve My Health When Strong <u>Lung-Lung</u> Are Causing Problems

This is one of the most unique and least-researched organ body systems. This body system is very delicate and should be taken care of with utmost care. Otherwise, the lifespan will abruptly be shortened.

Follow these recommendations if you have strong Lung organs already built in, and your life cycle is currently giving you extra of this organ energy and causing health issues.

See Chapter 3, "Strong Lung-Lung," to see if you are experiencing the listed symptoms.

Step 1 Avoid all foods from the Lung food list.

Avoid wifi routers and living near substations and cell towers.

Eat from the food lists of the following organs in the percentage indicated, per serving.

Stomach 25%
Liver 30%
Heart 30%
Kidney 15%

Until your body system is brought into balance, your past habits will try to unbalance you on continual basis. Do not eat items that will cause imbalance in your body. For quite some time, you will have to fight to stay balanced. However, it will give you greater return on your health. However, this will be up to you. It's always your choice.

Step 2 Eat bitter tasting foods for your heart.

Eat lamb and drink green tea, coffee, hot cocoa, ginseng daily. It will take much more time to balance than other organs. Think of a large pile of sturdy metal that you want to fashion into a good sword. It will take much pounding and work to make a fine sword out of the metal heap. However, it will be worth it in the end.

Once you decide to do it, you will accomplish it. You have strong lung power to see you through and get it done. When you are quick to anger or become impatient, acknowledge it and remind yourself that the pile of metal inside you is not yet refined.

The following recipes are special dishes for this body type.

**Use 1 tbsp of Chinese black bean paste by Chung Jung Won for stir fried vegetables or stew.

(Strong Lung-Lung, continued)

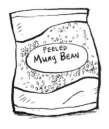

Tips on Mung Bean and Millet Pancakes

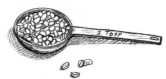

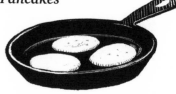

You can find peeled split mung beans online or in Asian grocery stores.

They are tiny and yellow in color.

The batter should be similar to regular pancake batter. Make sure the pan is hot and there's enough oil when you start.

Mung Bean and Millet Pancake

Ingredients:
- 2 cups peeled mung beans
- 1/2 cup of Indian millet
- 2 medium potatoes
- 1 cup dried cranberries, or 1 1/2 cup fresh/frozen cranberries
- 1/3 cup tapioca
- 1 egg
- 2 tsp good quality salt
- olive and sunflower seed oil

Directions:
1. Rinse and soak the peeled mung beans and the millet in 2–3 cups of warm water for 4 hours.
2. Add into the blender/food processor, the soaked mung beans, millet, potatoes, egg, salt, cranberries, tapioca, and enough water to just cover the ingredients. Blend to fine consistency.
3. Pour several tbsp of oil on to a hot pan, and ladle in the bean mixture to make small–medium sized pancakes. Flip once the edges turn golden brown.
4. If the bean batter is too watery, you can add flour for better consistency. If you add other items, it will change the medicinal property of this dish.
5. Huckleberries are a good match to eat with this pancake for this body type.
6. Eat with cranberry juice.

How often should I eat this pancake?

It should be eaten daily. **You will need to eat extra starting January 2021 to January 2022.**

It will calm your body and you won't be as quick to anger. You will feel kinder, with more energy, clarity and improved muscle and joint powers.

Lamb Stew

Ingredients:
- 1 lb. of lamb stew meat with fat trimmed off
- 3 small potatoes, diced
- 1 onion, diced
- 1 sweet yam, diced
- 1 medium carrot, diced
- 2 cups of cabbage, diced
- 2–3 cups of water
- salt or soup soy sauce/guk ganjang
- crushed walnuts, pecans as garnish
- perilla seed powder if you can find it

Directions:
1. Boil the stew meat and rinse the fat/grease off before transferring just the meat to a large pot or a slow cooker. (For slow cooker, dump everything in and cook for 6 hrs)
2. Add all the vegetables to the pot and pour in water
3. Bring to boil and then reduce heat and simmer for 1.5–2 hours.
4. Add salt and soy sauce to taste, 30 minutes before finishing.
5. Add a spoonful of crushed walnuts/pecans/perilla seed powder into the stew bowl and enjoy.
6. Eat with cranberry juice.

How often should I eat lamb?

(1) Eat this once daily for 2 weeks. (2) Reduce to 3–4 times a week for 3–6 months, depending on the severity of your condition. (3) Then reduce to once a week until it's no long needed. Your intensity will mellow out, with you becoming less impatient, and able to find more room to listen to others as you continue.

The following is another lamb option.

Lamb with Sweet Fruit Sauce

Ingredients:
- package of lamb meat from Costco, around $20–$34, fat removed
- ginger, thumb-sized peeled

Sauce ingredients:
- 1 cup of apricot fresh/dried
- 2 green apples
- 2 tbsp honey
- 1 tsp salt
- 1 cup dried cranberries
- 1 cup cabbage, diced

Directions:
1. Place defatted lamb meat into a large pot/pressure cooker with the ginger.
2. Cook the meat thoroughly.
3. Once finished cooking, remove from the pot and let it cool.
4. Cut into 1/2 inch slices.

Sauce Directions:
1. Put all the ingredients into a medium pot and bring to boil.
2. Reduce heat to medium low and cook for 30 min. to an hour. Make sure it doesn't boil over.
3. Once done, spoon over two slices of lamb and enjoy. You can also bake this in the oven for 30 min. at 350 degrees for more glazed lamb dish.
4. Eat with your choice of fresh vegetables and an optional 1-2 slices of bread.
5. Eat with cranberry juice.

(Strong Lung-Lung, continued)

At first, you may not like the smell of lamb, but it will get easier and you will find a way to remove the smell from the meat.

Your body will take this food in and will be completely absorbed without any heartburn or indigestion. You will also get hungry very soon afterward. Why? Because your body needed it yesterday. For medicinal purpose, you only need two slices to work. If you eat more than that during a single meal, your body might waste the rest. Wait 2–3 hours before eating another serving if you must. The body will take it in and use it.

Until your body system is brought into balance, your past habits will try to unbalance you on continual basis. Do not eat items that will cause imbalance in your body. For quite some time, you will have to fight to stay balanced. However, it will give you greater return on your health. However, this will be up to you. It's always your choice.

As your eating habits change, you will notice that you eat less of other things such as snacks because you feel generally satisfied. As a consequence, you may notice your grocery bill going down after several weeks.

After a few days or a few weeks, there should be noticeable improvement. Continue to take the beneficial foods until you reach a point of no discomfort.

You will return to better health conditions as if you had always been this healthy. And because a properly functioning body feels very natural and normal, and your body has nothing to complain about, you may not notice the changes as much. However, if you take note of your condition on a daily basis, you will recognize the improvements that you've already made.

***To expedite your health journey, create a virtue account by donating your time, talents, and/or money to help people in need once your body system gets better. If you are already doing that, increase the amount you do without thinking about having done it. Basically, don't let the left hand know what the right hand has done. The return on your investment will be greater than you might think.

If this is not possible, take five minutes from your day to reflect and be thankful, praying or sending out thoughts of good will to all humanity. It will elevate you and all of humanity.

***Please note**: to reduce the risk of foodborne illness, it's important to cook the lamb meat thoroughly (well done) before consuming.

How to Improve My Health When Strong
<u>Lung-Stomach</u> or <u>Stomach-Lung</u> Are Causing Problems

Follow these recommendations if you have strong Lung and Stomach organs already built in, and your life cycle is currently giving you an excess of these organ energies and causing health issues.

See Chapter 3, "Strong Lung-Stomach"/"Strong Stomach-Lung," to see if you are experiencing the listed symptoms.

Step 1 Avoid all foods from the Lung and Stomach food lists.

Avoid wifi routers and living near substations and cell towers.

Eat from the food lists of the following organs in the percentage indicated, per serving.

Liver 40%
Heart 40%
Kidney 20%

Until your body system is brought into balance, your past habits will try to unbalance you on continual basis. Do not eat items that will cause imbalance in your body. For quite some time, you will have to fight to stay balanced. However, it will give you greater return on your health. However, this will be up to you. It's always your choice.

Step 2 Take in lamb, green tea, coffee, hot cocoa, or ginseng daily.

**Use 1 tbsp of Chinese black bean paste by Chung Jung Won for stir-fried vegetables or stew.

Take in beans, avocado, and 100% cranberry juice.

The following are special dishes for this body type.

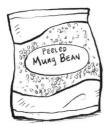 *Tips on Mung Bean and Millet Pancakes*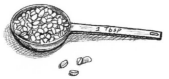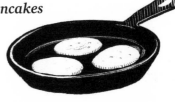

You can find peeled split mung beans online or in Asian grocery stores.

They are tiny and yellow in color.

The batter should be similar to regular pancake batter. Make sure the pan is hot and there's enough oil when you start.

Mung Bean and Millet Pancake

Ingredients:
- 2 cups peeled mung beans
- 1/2 cup of Indian millet
- 1/4 cup dried cranberries
- 1 egg
- 2 tsp good quality salt
- olive and sunflower seed oil

Directions:
1. Rinse and soak the peeled mung beans and the millet in 2–3 cups of warm water for 4 hours.
2. Add into the blender/food processor, the soaked mung beans, millet, egg, salt, and enough water to just cover the ingredients. Blend to fine consistency.
3. Mix in the cranberries into the batter.
4. Pour several tbsp of oil on to a hot pan, and ladle in the bean mixture to make small–medium sized pancakes. Flip once the edges turn golden brown.
5. If the bean batter is too watery, you can add flour for better consistency. If you add other items, it will change the medicinal property of this dish.
6. Huckleberries or extra amounts of cranberries are a good match to eat with this pancake for this body type.
7. Eat with cranberry juice.

How often should I eat this pancake?

It should be eaten daily. **You will need to eat extra starting January 2021 to January 2022.**

It will calm your body and you won't be as quick to anger. You will feel kinder, with more energy, clarity and improved muscle and joint powers.

Chicken and Clam Soup

Ingredients:

- 2 chicken breasts, diced/ sliced.
- 1 can of clams/clam juice
- 3 kombu/seaweed pieces 2"x2"
- 1/2 cup of dried mushrooms, sliced
- 2 tsp salt/2 tbsp soup soy sauce
- 2 eggs
- 3 cups of water

Directions:

1. Trim the fat off the chicken breast.
2. On a hot pan, lightly sear the chicken breasts on both sides.
3. Dice or slice the chicken breasts to bite-sized pieces.
4. In a large pot, combine chicken, clams, seaweed, mushrooms, salt/soup soy sauce, and water, cooking for 20–30 minutes.
5. Add beaten eggs to the soup right before turning off the stove.

How often should I eat this soup?

Eat this daily. In a few days to a week, your intensity will mellow out. You will become less impatient, and able to find more room to listen to others as you continue. Afterward, reduce to 2–3 times a week.

It's a different eating habit and taste, but your body will take this food in and will be completely absorbed without any heartburn or indigestion. You will also get hungry very soon afterward. Why? Because your body needed it yesterday. Eat this 2–3 times a day at the beginning. For medicinal purpose, you only need two slices for it to work. If you eat more than that during a single meal, your body might waste the rest. Wait 2–3 hours before eating another serving. The body will take it in and use it.

Until your body system is brought into balance, your past habits will try to unbalance you on continual basis. Do not eat items that will cause imbalance in your body. For quite some time, you will have to fight to stay balanced. However, it will give you greater return on your health. However, this will be up to you. It's always your choice.

As your eating habits change, you will notice that you eat less of other things such as snacks because you feel generally satisfied. As a consequence, you may notice your grocery bill going down after several weeks.

After a few days or a few weeks, there should be noticeable improvement. Continue to take the beneficial foods until you reach a point of no discomfort.

You will return to better health conditions as if you had always been this healthy. And because a properly functioning body feels very natural and normal, and your body has nothing to complain about, you may not notice the changes as much. However, if you take note of your condition on a daily basis, you will recognize the improvements that you've already made.

***To expedite your health journey, create a virtue account by donating your time, talents, and/or money to help people in need once your body system gets better. If you are already doing that, increase the amount you do without thinking about having done it. Basically, don't let the left hand know what the right hand has done. The return on your investment will be greater than you might think.

If this is not possible, take five minutes from your day to reflect and be thankful, praying or sending out thoughts of good will to all humanity. It will elevate you and all of humanity.

How to Improve My Health When Strong <u>Stomach-Stomach</u> Are Causing Problems

Follow these recommendations if you have a strong Stomach organ already built in, and your life cycle is currently giving you an excess of this organ energy and causing health issues.

See Chapter 3, "Strong Stomach-Stomach," to see if you are experiencing the listed symptoms.

Step 1   Avoid all foods from the Stomach food list. This is a must.

Eat from the food lists of the following organs in the percentage indicated, per serving.

Kidney 35%
Heart 20%
Liver 30%
Lung 15%

Until your body system is brought into balance, your past habits will try to unbalance you on continual basis. Do not eat items that will cause imbalance in your body. For quite some time, you will have to fight to stay balanced. However, it will give you greater return on your health. However, this will be up to you. It's always your choice.

Step 2   This is an inexpensive way to cool down the inner temperature and soothe the system. This soup will instantly make you feel more comfortable both physically and emotionally.

Seaweed and Bone Marrow Soup

Ingredients:
- 1/2 cup dried seaweed, cut into 2" lengths
- 1/2 cup of dried mushrooms
- 1 can of clams/clam juice
- 3 scallops
- 1 squid
- 1/2 cup of radish, thinly sliced
- 1 cup beef bone broth
- 1 tsp sesame seed oil
- good quality salt/soup soy sauce (guk-ganjang)
- mung bean sprouts (optional)
- 1/4 cup crushed pine nuts or walnuts (optional)

Directions:
1. Soak the dried seaweed in warm water for 10 min. Rinse and put into a large pot with 7 cups of water and bring to boil.
2. Add mushrooms, clams/clam juice, sesame oil, walnuts, scallops, squid, and radishes.
3. Season with salt/soup soy sauce and let it cook for additional 15 min.
4. Add mung bean sprouts 2 min. prior to serving (optional).
5. Add a spoonful of crushed pine nuts to the bowl before eating (optional).

(Strong Stomach-Stomach, continued)

*Eating seaweed and cucumber salad also highly recommended.

How often should I eat the seaweed soup?

It should be eaten daily.

After a few days or a few weeks, there should be noticeable improvement. Continue to take the beneficial foods until you reach a point of no discomfort.

You will return to better health conditions as if you had always been this healthy. And because a properly functioning body feels very natural and normal, and your body has nothing to complain about, you may not notice the changes as much. However, if you take note of your condition on a daily basis, you will recognize the improvements that you've already made.

***To expedite your health journey, create a virtue account by donating your time, talents, and/or money to help people in need once your body system gets better. If you are already doing that, increase the amount you do without thinking about having done it. Basically, don't let the left hand know what the right hand has done. The return on your investment will be greater than you might think.

If this is not possible, take five minutes from your day and take that time to reflect and be thankful, praying or sending out thoughts of good will to all humanity. It will elevate you and all of humanity.

Chapter 7

External Energies

External Energies Entering Our Body

External energies can be anything: another person, a thing, a thought that pops up, weather, place, the universe, or anything other than what we have internally.

A prime example is the Covid-19 pandemic that we are all presently experiencing. This is both an unprecedented and unexpected global event that has taken many lives and leaves the future uncertain because we don't know the cause or the cure. The virus has altered our lives forever, changing the way we live and work. The external energy has affected us both internally and externally.

There are many contributing factors that goes with the Covid-19 pandemic. Here, we will discuss the yearly external energy changes that affect us.

Presently, what the external energy is bringing in is extremely cold, icy water. It's not normal icy water. This extreme cold penetrates into our body system to shock, jolt, freeze, damage, and alter our internal systems. Some body structures are not equipped to deal with an event like this.

This cycle comes only once every 60 years. In the olden days, if people made it through their 61st birthday, it was considered a blessing and was celebrated as a special milestone. Nowadays, tremendous improvements in the way we live have allowed us to live well into our 80s. With some more changes, most of us will reach our 100s in the not too distant future.

This year's external changes are affecting just about everyone. Some are affected less than others, some are critically ill, and some are dying from it. This is especially true for those with the following organ types when they don't have other supporting organs to take care of the body: Stomach-Lung, Stomach-Heart, weak Liver, weak Kidney, Lung-Kidney, and strong Lungs .

Some organ systems are able to handle this extremely cold and icy water energy running through their system. However, it's tough at times.

Who will most likely make it through okay?

The people with strong Heart-Lung, strong Heart-Kidney, and Heart-Liver will be the least to suffer.

If we learn to understand our body's system and how it signals, we can proactively protect ourselves and better weather through times like this. When we have an unequipped body system facing a virus like Covid-19, we can at least prepare to slow it down or stop it, and hang on until help becomes available.

It's a roller coaster of energies this year, where even the well maintained organ body systems will be affected. This is especially a terrible time for those with low to weak immune systems and the people with the following organ types:

Strong Stomach-Kidney
Strong Stomach-Heart
Strong Stomach-Lung
Strong Stomach-Stomach

Strong Lung-Kidney
Strong Lung-Heart
Strong Lung-Lung
Strong Lung-Stomach

And those who have:
Weak Kidneys
Weak Heart
Weak Liver
Weak Lungs

The first damaged group will be those with weak Kidneys (water tank is empty) and weak Heart. The second damaged group will be those with weak Liver (no life energy left to continue). The third damaged group will be those with strong Lungs and Lung-Kidney organs (without support of Heart and Liver, they will suffer greatly). Strong Lungs plus the intense external Lung energy overwhelms the Liver system. On the other side, those with weak lungs suffer as well because without established lung capacity, they won't be able to handle the incoming intensity of the external Lung energy.

However, for those who are aware and are trying to maintain their health by harmonizing their organ systems, they can have a wonderful and prosperous time. And those who need this icy water energy in their system, like Heart-Kidney, and Heart-Liver, will also prosper. These body types are able to handle the external energy of 2020 and 2021 much better than any other group. The virus can come in but these body systems melt it away as soon as it comes in.

The people with their five organs somewhat in harmony may be touched by the virus but it will pass away quickly. Some may not even know it even came in. And as a consequence, some won't understand what all the fuss is about when it comes to Covid-19. For whatever reasons, even now there are some who assume that the news of countless deaths from the pandemic is fake news and dismiss the seriousness of this virus. For them, this pandemic won't be real until they run into their own organ deficiencies and suffer a devastating and unexpected illness themselves. And they will suffer greatly unless they understand how to take care of their body's needs.

When these naysayers finally become sick, those who have already suffered and survived the Covid-19 will have very little compassion to give them in return. This disconnect between people during times like this will continue until we all realize that everyone is built differently and therefore will get sick differently and will require different treatments.

For those of us who understand the seriousness of this pandemic after having experienced it and know what it's like, it is good to remember that we, too, were clueless when Covid-19 first arrived. We should give those who remain ignorant our understanding because someday they will understand it as well.

In the past as in the present, illnesses like this one, which don't neatly fit into a uniform box of explanations, have baffled scientists and doctors. Why does one person do okay while another dies from it? And when they come up with a treatment, why does it work for one group and not for the other? Ultimately, they have to go with the treatment that works for the majority of the group and put everyone into that box.

We need specialists who can treat those who don't fit into that box. Those who don't respond to standard medical treatments are left with very few options for treating their condition. They require qualified specialists who can provide them with the specialized services that they need. And they are willing to pay for those services.

Can an external energy change my moods and eating habits?

Yes.

Can external energies change how I feel about other people?

Yes. Our body is affected by internal and external energies. If the external changes happen to give us better internal harmony, we will be perceived by others in more positive light. In the same way, if the other person is receiving positive support from the external energies, we tend to think of that person in a more favorable light. If the external energies happen to be negative for us or the other person, the favorable impression shifts to the unfavorable. Like or dislike, it shifts with the energies. However, there are minds that are unmoved by any of these energy changes. Ultimately, that's where we want to be. We want to be free from energy politics.

How will the external energy changes of 2020 and 2021 affect our body system?

From December 2019 to November 2020, it will be a terrible time for those with strong Lungs, weak Heart, weak Kidney, and weak Liver. Without Heart, Liver and Kidney support, it will be a difficult year for these body systems.

Let us observe and investigate the next 12 years for the adjustment of our body, and a chance to maneuver the incoming energies to better protect ourselves. We can alter the outcome by preparing and protecting our health, money, power, fame, dignity, and longevity by supporting the weaker organ systems.

The external energy that we are experiencing actually started back in December of 2019. Normally, the changes occur in January, but this is subject to the changes in the earth's axis.

What are the effects for the above body systems?

When this extremely cold and icy water enters the body system, the body goes into shock. This is because the body was never ready to accept in such huge magnitude this type of energy. It overwhelms the body system by freezing and shocking it as it disables the heart and the circulatory system in a very short time. The body has no time to make adjustments to deal with the incoming change.

How long will it last?

It is strongest at the beginning of the cycle, and the impact eventually slows. Regardless, the energy remains and affects our body system from December 2019 to November 2020 and from December 2020 to November 2021. Though the same effect will continue into 2021 with only a slight difference, it will be a deadlier year for some. Because our body system has suffered a great deal of damage already from the previous year, it won't have time to recover before the next strong impact of 2021. This is especially so for those with strong Lungs, weak Liver, weak Heart, and weak Kidneys. Some of our body systems will not be ready to endure the extended onslaught of the 2021 external energies without the support of our weaker/troubled organs.

When is my cycle of change?

Observe hourly, daily, monthly, and yearly changes within our system.

Every ten years, a major new cycle of energies enters and affects each and every individual with that energy. And all of us are in different individual phases. We like it when the energy feels good and we don't like it when if feels bad. What is the use of liking or disliking the good, the bad, and the ugly, which are just regular parts of our lives? Just acknowledge that it's there and make adjustments accordingly for ourselves. It's not worth choosing one over the other because, soon, something else will show up to disrupt our opinions. So, acknowledge it and let go without judgment. Clinging to our ideas causes blockage to our growth and we end up going through unnecessary suffering. When we acknowledge and let go, we gain the momentum to move forward with life that is stress-free.

External energies that affect us.

When the incoming organ energies are something that our body needs, we are in luck. We will be elevated from the previous cycle and life will seem much easier, happier, and more prosperous.

Sometimes, the lucky cycle may continue, depending on the sequence of cycles. We are on a lucky path if the next one also supports our weak organs. However, this isn't a forever thing. Though we wish it could last forever, that's not how the universe runs. When the sequence changes, so does our luck, which ends with the cycle.

Can a cycle change my health, money, power, fame, dignity, and longevity?

They will absolutely change with the cycles. Some for the better, and some for the worse, depending on our organ systems.

Out of the Cycle of Health, Money, Power, Fame, and Dignity.

The following story is about a woman who claimed that she didn't know how she got so lucky before God suddenly took it all away from her.

I met her about 10 years ago. I was looking to hire a person for one my projects who happened to be an expert in an area that was not my strength. She seemed to have all the qualifications that I was looking for and maybe even more. Though she asked nicely, she demanded that our meeting take place in her town, which was two hours away. I thought, maybe she had what I was looking for, and if she was the right person, the trip would be worth it. I drove two hours to meet her at a diner. She was well dressed, attractive, maybe in her 60s, highly intelligent, and sophisticated. In the course of our conversation, she told me that she was one powerful diplomat's wife and that she had previously played a significant role in government connections. She had had everything at her finger tips, able to do as she pleased. That habit still remained with her even after all these years, and she continued to reminisce about that time. I asked her if she could do my project. She replied that she could.

We agreed to meet in the next couple of weeks to go forward with the project and talk over the details. She nicely demanded a $1,000 deposit to show that I was serious about this and to reserve her time exclusively for this project. All the meetings had to be in her town because she didn't travel out of the area. I had no problem with that. She had already prepared a contract, and I gave her a refundable deposit and agreed to meet the following week.

On our next meeting, I brought $100 worth of fine chocolates to give her. She had no warmth in her body system. In my eyes, she was like a flickering light that was ready to go out any time.

When I presented the chocolates to her, she uncharacteristically made a quick grab for it, asking how I had known that she liked high quality chocolates.

I gave her instructions on how to help herself and improve the condition of her health. We had a long conversation. I wanted to deliver my message to her as kindly and warmly as possible. This was no longer about the project. Rather, I had a deep and great concern for where she would likely end up in the very near future.

She knew where she had been and how she got to now, but she didn't know about the end game. I told her that the $1,000 deposit was my investment for her healing journey. Not knowing what was happening and being unable to take care of her body was not a good choice for her.

Being caught up in her anger, fear, sorrow, blame and disappointments throughout her life was not good. That wasn't all of her, but she had lost her life to it because she couldn't see herself beyond her emotional state. My offer of help touched her.

I suggested mending her relationship with her mother. She said that it couldn't be done even if she wanted to. The relationship was beyond repair and her mother didn't want anything to do with her. Each time they spoke, the conversation would quickly devolve into a blaming game. Now, there were no more talks.

Nevertheless, I told her to buy a thank-you card for her mother. And to tell her that she had been young and stupid, not knowing what she was doing. She was to tell her mother that she was sorry and hurting her was the last thing she had wanted to do. She had clung like a bratty child, and was unkind when her mother had asked for help. If her mother had the heart to forgive her, she wanted to learn from her how to be a considerate and loving daughter even at this late age.

When I finished, the woman became angry and demanded to know who had put me up to this. I told her, "It was you."

She wasn't expecting this. I told her some of her life stories as if I had been there. And I told her where she was, and where she was heading.

Eventually, something moved within her. After many tears and show of anger, she accepted my offer with gratitude. Then she revealed to me that on the morning of our first meeting, she had an unusual dream. She smiled and looked happy but didn't tell me what the dream was about, and I didn't ask. Perhaps, it was a dream connected to my offer.

Grateful, she wanted to do my project as her number-one priority. I told her that my project had to wait until she recovered.

I told her how the cycle of energies ran. God hadn't taken away her glorious life in the past. It was simply the next cycle that she was on, and she had not been equipped to deal with it. She neither had the knowledge nor the body to support her through the change, so she had no choice but to fall as low as she had. But this time, she could make improvements. When the next difficult cycle hits, she could fall and land gracefully instead of crashing and burning. This information somehow brought calm to her.

If a cycle provides excess of that energy which we have built in already in our body system, it can be difficult. Things won't work in our favor for that cycle or the next, if they are similar. That may not be what we want, but it's going to come anyway for a period of time. But we can do something to reduce its impact.

This is not about fairness, or liking or disliking.

I told her that she had co-created the program that she was in. Perhaps she had done it to learn something. Perhaps it was for working on a certain project or to build a bridge for the next level of her journey. That woke her up and lit her like a bright star. Somehow, this had given her clarity on what she was looking for. I didn't ask what it was because I didn't need to know.

Sometimes, just the internal energy itself, or more often in combination with the external energies, can create harmony or disharmony in a person.

Next, understand what external energies are affecting our body throughout 2020 while it is still fresh and current.

Coronavirus and the Fear of the Unknown

In March of 2020, I received a call from someone I knew. He said the doctor had just confirmed that he had the Covid-19. He had been sick for ten days and was continuing to get worse. As far as the doctor or the hospital was concerned, his symptoms weren't severe enough for him to be admitted to the hospital. He was told to stay home and just take care of it. Unless he had severe breathing problems, he couldn't be hospitalized.

He said it was like they were telling him to go away and just wait to die because they couldn't help him. Yes, death was certainly possible, but they were hoping that he would live through it and recover at home like the others. The doctors didn't know how to help him as they had no known remedy to treat the illness.

With the hospital rejecting him, he had no place to turn. He had been suffering for ten days with the symptoms continuing to get worse, and yet he wasn't sick enough to be admitted. Fear and uncertainty gripped him as he faced an unknown future alone. It felt terribly hopeless and unfamiliar.

He described his physical symptoms. There was weakness, body aches and pains all over, with a periodic sharp pain in his chest and heart. He was unable to lie down or sit comfortably due to the pain in his shoulder blade area, and was having diarrhea-like symptoms, dry mouth, foggy mind, no appetite, and no direction.

He had never experienced anything like this before. He was in his mid 60s with a strong Stomach-Heart organ system.

"Is this how I am going to die?" he said over the phone. It sounded like he was talking more to himself.

The fear of the unknown, and him possibly dying at any moment triggered a great fear inside of him. He wasn't sure if he would wake up the next day to see the morning light. That was the pandemic fear growing inside of him, leading him into a dark thought process. That wasn't a wise path to follow.

I gave him instructions for making Spicy Chicken Soup, and doing sun meditations and hot-and-cold shower. These were simple remedies within his reach, but it would be up to him to follow.

He followed everything as directed, and by the fourth day he was doing well enough to get off the soup and the hot and cold shower. Now recovered, he continues to take care of himself by eating the foods needed by his organs and doing periodic sun meditations.

How Do the Yearly Changes in External Energy Affect Our Body System?

The following information helps us understand how our body is affected by the external energy sources and what we can do to cope through the maneuvering of our body system.

Let's start with 2020, the year that has severe energy fluctuations for every body type. Again, it is extremely terrible for people with strong Lungs, weak Heart, weak Liver, and weak Kidneys. The body is unable to bear all this cold energy but it all depends on other factors that come into play. This external energy is harsh icy water that penetrates our body system without mercy. But it is what it is and will do what it is scheduled to do. All we can do is to prepare, or not prepare.

See "Strong Lung-Kidney" in "Organs and their Symptoms," Chapter 3. The severity will be three times as strong.

Normal delivery for each external energy changes will come strong at the beginning, and then taper off until it reaches the end of the cycle where it will be 20% to 30% weaker than when it first started. Though the initial damage won't be significant at first, the damage will be there, nevertheless. This is the normal situation. When the following year is similar to the current one, it gets much more damaging and that is what we will be facing next.

We help our body to maintain and add more buffers to our system by supplying triple the normal amount of the foods that our body system requires. This provides cushion to lessen the damaging impact of the oncoming external energy for those who are affected.

The impact we felt from the 2020 external energy felt ten times worse because, internally, we were having a great ride with abundance of material things, dressed in light summer clothes and enjoying the warmth. We were completely enjoying ourselves in the energy that was present while being completely oblivious to the impending superstorm of ice.

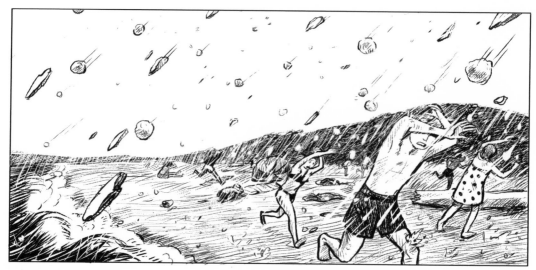

When it arrived, all of a sudden we found ourselves in a hail storm with ice chunks falling from the sky. As we got pelted by the giant frozen ice pellets, we were running around in our bathing suits panicking and not understanding what was happening. Some died from the impact and some suffered injury. Everyone was scrambling to get to their cars, and those who made it sighed with relief at finding shelter. But what they didn't realize was that the impact of this storm had already infiltrated their body system in a way that couldn't be easily shaken off.

This event is a part of a natural cycle, as well as unnatural creations, of a universal system. It's not good or bad, or something to be angry about. It's something that we weather through because we are part of the universe. Our own body system is a small version of that universe. We are all connected and all the systems are running at the same time.

Did we know of the coming impact?

Some may have been aware of the incoming impact but they were unable to describe it in full until they had experienced it themselves, due to other factors playing a role. Regardless, the event takes place whether we know it or not. Most of us were caught unprepared after having a great time the previous year. If we had known and actually prepared for this event, it would have helped in minimizing the impact.

The external energies of 2020 will prove to be deadly for certain organ body types while causing suffering for others. And some will benefit from it. Regardless, it will all stop with the passing of this cycle.

How Can I Mitigate the Effects of
External Energies on Our Body System?

The following are some good ways of alleviating the effects of external energies on our organ systems.

How to protect my memory system and prevent Alzeheimer's during this cycle.

Our current cycle (2020) and the next coming cycle (2021) will impact and weaken our Liver system and our memory system like no other time in history.

<u>For those with strong Lung energy</u>: Strong Lung energy continues to chop and damage the Liver system. Supplying the body system with enough Liver energy is recommended. Most importantly, avoid all foods for Lungs. This body tends to favor/demand Lung foods, which will be terrible for memory health.

<u>For those who lack Liver energy</u>: Following the food list for Liver is recommended.

<u>For those who lack Kidney energy</u>: Some organ types, like strong Heart-Stomach, will need to supply a healthy amount of Kidney energy to other organs because these cycles will increasingly use up the life energy of the person.

Strong Heart/Stomach types tend to withdraw Kidney energy without resupplying their Kidney system. This is not recommended.

Following the food list for Kidney and Liver is recommended.

How can I tell if I am lacking or have excess in Kidney/Lung organs?

People who lack Kidney energy (Strong Heart-Stomach type people) are usually outgoing, mingle with others easily, and are sweet.

Strong Lung organ type people are usually very direct, bossy, cold, don't like to be told what to do, or chitchat.

If the organ imbalance is at beginning stages, the condition will improve with Kidney and Liver foods.

If the organ imbalance is severe, it will take a while to reach the critical point with the Kidney and Liver foods. It all depends on each individual and how their body is built.

How do I remove the extremely cold ice cubes out of my system?

There's much work to be done. It is very important to melt the ice cubes out of the body. Otherwise, it will continue to flow throughout our body system and create problems for a long time. We have to find a way to melt it away. Even though we may feel fine at times, think what happens when a frostbite goes untreated. Something eventually shrivels and dies.

Following the recipe for Spicy Chicken Soup, taking hot-and-cold showers, and sunbathing in the morning will help with melting the ice cubes. Depending on the severity and whether the cold energy is still coming in, it may take time to completely melt them out of our system. Since this cold external energy is continuing to come in, those with affected body systems will have to work diligently to make it through until November of 2021.

Spicy Chicken Soup

Ingredients:
- 2 chicken breasts (organic if available), rinsed
- 1 tsp salt
- 7 cups of water
- 1/2 cup of sake (optional)
- 5–7 dry hot peppers (Do not substitute with any hot sauce. It will work differently.)
- 1/2 cup dried shitake mushrooms
- 1 onion
- 2 cups cabbage, sliced thinly
- 1–2 tsp salt
- 1 medium ginger, peeled and sliced
- 2 bundles of green onions/scallions, washed well and cut into 3" lengths
- 2 green apples, diced
- hot chili pepper powder
- crushed walnut or cashew (optional)

Directions:
1. Boil the rinsed chicken, adding 1 tsp of salt. When finished, chop the chicken meat and discard water.
2. In a large pot, combine 7 cups of water, chicken, sake, dry hot peppers, dried shitake mushrooms, onion, cabbage, salt, ginger, and green onions and bring to boil on high heat.
3. Reduce heat to medium-low and simmer for 30–40 minutes.
4. Before turning off the heat, stir in the chopped apples and cover with lid.
5. Serve in mid-size bowl, <u>adding tbsp of hot chili pepper powder</u> and crushed walnuts/cashews.

How often: Eat three bowls a day until the whole pot is finished. Adding that spoonful of chili pepper to the bowl is key.

At first, our body may seem to reject this dish because we're not used to it. Also, the invaders in our body system will keep hinting that we don't want to eat the soup. With the soup in our body system, they may not be able to stay long and do damage, so they will fight to keep the soup out.

After two servings, we will feel better but not all the way. Continue to take the soup. The pot of soup should take 2–3 days to finish. If you don't like or are allergic to some of the ingredients, cook without them. However, keep in mind that every ingredient serves a purpose in the soup.

Cook and eat again as it becomes necessary.
This spicy chicken soup can be beneficial until January 2022.

What's the benefit?

The soup will provide warmth to the body and the tools to fight and melt away the icy water particles in the body system.

Hot-and-Cold Shower

Taking a hot-and-cold shower is recommended for jump-starting healthy circulation in the body and expelling the cold energy out of the body system. It's definitely not everyone's cup of tea and it may feel impossible, but it is effective and will expedite the process of kicking out the icy energy from the body.

Use fresh bedding and clothing with each hot-and-cold shower and allow air and sunlight to circulate throughout the rooms from time to time.

Hot-and-cold shower	1. Wash hair first, and do the following from the neck down. 2. Hot water for 3 minutes 3. Warm water for 2 minutes 4. Cold water for 2 minutes 5. Hot water for 2 minutes 6. Cold water for 2 minutes 7. Hot water for 2 minutes 8. Cold water for 30 seconds to finish 9. Dry hair and put on warm clothing and socks to let the body sweat and let the cold icy water exit out of the body. Stay warm for at least 1 hour. Dry hair is a must.

A hot sauna will also work. To finish up the sauna, take a cold shower for 1 minute and then put on warm clothing and warm socks after that. Dry hair is a must.

Along with daily food intake for weak organs, by the second day, the body should feel better. By the third day, the body will feel much better. On the fourth day, the body should have recovered by 90%. Continue until body feels fully recovered.

The soup, the morning sunbathing, and the hot-and-cold shower may take some getting used to, but if one is willing, they will help the body heal and get this problem out of our system. They are inexpensive and doable tools for staying healthy.

Morning Sunbathing or Walking Sun Meditation

For those who can tolerate the sun, taking in the right amount of morning sun for about 30–60 minutes daily will really strengthen our immune system and our cells. Sitting outside under indirect sunlight will also help. However, doing this without also supplying the body with enough Kidney energy can be dangerous. Those who refuse to take Kidney energy shouldn't do sunbathing. And drinking just water by itself won't be enough.

Observe, know, and investigate through our body system to learn to take care of our body. Do not look for something to blame. Just understand and observe. Some may take only a short time to understand and be able to practice taking care of their body. And for some, it make take several years or a lifetime to fully understand and remedy. It all depends on the information system created by our habits.

If we have stored relevant information from the past, it will be easier to learn and understand. With a lot of stored information, we can pick up quickly, making connections as we go along. If we have no such stored information, we will need to learn the basic ABC's and build our knowledge base to use now and in the future.

Of course, we also have the never-ending parade of thoughts that comes out of our heads, all the guessing and accumulated information that we have picked up from here and there. We can certainly make our decisions from this place, but we've traveled down this road already.

Turn a question within.

We have a wisdom source that isn't from our head with its guessing and accumulated information. This source is in our conscience, and that's where we want to go. We will receive a surprise answer from within to give us confidence in its power and the knowledge to follow. Some of us may have already realized this. That would be a very good thing.

Once all our organs connect and get well, we will have a more peaceful mind that's able to grasp and know more than before. But until then, it will only be our logic's dreamland.

Right now, we can only know through a part of a body system that is not fully connected and energized. Once the body functions as a fully connected and energized system, the extent of the knowledge, freedom, and wisdom that will be available to us will be unfathomable.

Learning to nurture ourselves means that we are heading towards that wisdom stage.

What happens when we turn within to get answers?

When all the conditions are met, we will no longer be subject to whatever problems we are facing. We know that it's happening, but we're much less affected by it. Life continues to go on whether we participate in it or not. Our bad life drama is the same way. Once we follow our inner wisdom and the body conditions are met, the bad drama will have less effect on us or may even disappear altogether, with or without notice.

Our five organs' sense of sight, smell, hearing, taste, and touch provide delightful information based on their expertise. However, getting us out of our mess is not their function. As the owners of our body, we have both the responsibility and authority to take good care of it with due diligence.

We know this logically, right? But if we observe closely, we should notice that we follow our senses and feelings without question, as if they are our infallible guide or guiding principle.

Let's learn to direct a question within and recognize the answer that arises from within.

"What is it?"
"What's causing it?"

Once we put a question to ourselves, an answer may arise from within us in the form of hints, signals, images, or dreams that show us what to do. All living things have this ability. It is the wisdom that arises from within, the ultimate truth. This mind has no boundaries or restrictions. It has no concept of good or bad, and does not swing from side to side. This mind exists when we eat, work, sleep, etc. It appears when we rely on it. This nature exists so that we can exist in this moment, and it will exist eons after this moment.

We don't have to try to be kind, pure, pretty, powerful, principled, etc. It all comes naturally with a harmonized organ system, without all the roller coaster of mental and emotional plays.

Try it and see whether it is correct or not.

For example, let's say a child has a fever of 20–30 degrees Celsius during winter and is requesting watermelon. This is what the child's body is craving. What do we do? Do we tell the child logically and calmly that we don't eat watermelon in the middle of freezing winter, especially when one has a high fever?

By doing this, we are basically telling the child that this is a crazy idea. Even though we didn't say this explicitly, this is what we are delivering to the child—that the child's need/request is crazy. The child's internal wisdom has received the message loud and clear and will be reluctant to share next time. And from this experience, the child will go through unnecessary suffering because of our logic.

The request for the watermelon sounds illogical to our thoughts. But some of us will take the child's request seriously, especially if we know the child to be genuine, and run to the grocery store to purchase whatever watermelon is available in middle of winter. This is how we honor and trust the child, and show our love. Once the child eats the amount of watermelon the child needs, the fever goes down and the child's body returns to normal.

How do we explain this logically? We can't, so we lie and cover it up with excuses to save our egos.

The child identified what the body was craving, made a request, and it was answered. The same thing applies to us adults. When our inside tells us that we need watermelon in the middle of winter to remedy an imbalance in our body, our logic pushes it way because it sounds illogical. If we continue to do things from the logic's point of view, we won't be hearing much message from inside. It will only answer when we show that we are serious about listening.

Once we are indeed serious about listening and actually act on the messages/directions, we will receive more precise answers from within. The answers are very subtle, so we have to be awake to hear it. It will be more a whisper than a loud clap of thunder. With this, we will know what to do to fill the holes in our body system. And, we will find freedom and wisdom.

Observation of the Next
Twelve-Year Cycle

Let's observe and investigate the next twelve years and see how they will influence us physically, emotionally, and spiritually.

2021: It's the Reign of the Strong Heartless Lung.

It's a slightly different pattern but the energies from 2020 will continue on. This makes it extremely difficult for people with strong Lungs, Lung-Kidney, and Lung-Stomach, and those with weak Liver, Kidney and Heart.

Frequent bursts of anger will rise out of nowhere and everywhere, for no reason and for every reason. It will be easily triggered and very difficult to control at times.

Before acting out in anger, drink a glass of orange/grape juice, and follow directions for taking in food for the Heart, Liver, and Kidney.

Energywise, it's a harsh and ruthless winter. It is time for chopping, removing, reorganizing, and reestablishing of the grounds for the beginning of Lung's reign. This energy will only last a year, but its ruthless and heartless power will feel like it will go on forever.

If we act on it without considering the consequences, we will pay a heavy price for it. Whether we benefit or not from these energies, we will be affected by them. For the entire year, refrain from acting on this ruthless and heartless energies. By choosing not to follow these terrible energies, it will give us 11 or more years of freedom from it.

Those with strong Heart-Kidney will benefit a great deal. Others may feel they got the bad end of the stick. No blame is needed. It's a cycle that we all face. Careful intake of the right foods will minimize and reduce impact, and will carry us to the cycle of Spring, where warm and gentle nurturing awaits in 2022.

Observe and see whether this is true or not. Once we are serious about listening, we will receive more precise answers from within.

2022: It's pre-Spring time.
Nature/universe offers nurturing after two very difficult years.
However, it is a harsh time for people with weak Stomach, weak Heart, and weak Lungs.

2023: It's the time of cold Spring energy.
It's a harsh time for people with weak Heart, weak Stomach, weak Lungs, and strong Lungs.

2024: It's the time of rising Life energy.
It's a harsh time for those with weak Kidneys and strong Liver.

2025: It's the time of Spring flowers.
It's a harsh time for those with weak Kidneys, and occasionally for strong Lungs.

2026: It's the time of ultimate and extreme Fire.
It's a harsh time for those with weak Lungs, weak Kidneys, weak Liver, and strong Heart.

2027: It's the time of beautiful candlelight.
It's a harsh time for those with weak Kidneys and weak Lungs.

2028: It's the time of damp Autumn, and great business ventures.
It's a harsh time for those with weak Liver, weak Kidneys, weak Heart, and occasionally, for strong Lungs.

2029: It's the time of Golden Harvest.
It's a harsh time for those with weak Liver, weak Kidneys, strong Stomach, and occasionally for strong Lungs.

2030: It's the time of cold Autumn, after the harvest.
It's a harsh time for those with weak Liver, strong Lungs, weak Heart, weak Stomach.

2031: It's the time of harsh Winter.
It's terrible time for those with weak Heart, weak Stomach, weak Liver and weak Kidneys.

2032: It's the time for Winter of Winters, a new era of business.
It's a harsh time for those with weak Heart, weak Stomach, strong Lung, strong Kidneys, and strong Liver.

Did we learn and recognize the things that were happening to our body and make the necessary adjustments to remedy the symptoms?

If we didn't quite make the necessary adjustments, we may not be able to see the results of our work clearly. But nevertheless, we are still standing here.

For some, it may take only a short time, while for others it may take several years to a lifetime to fully understand and balance their body system. However, it will still be a shorter method than anything else for creating a harmonized body system.

Even with certain inner programs at work, it is important to maintain a proper body system. It won't be perfect, but it will be able to weather the inevitable storms that come our way. Most importantly, through this we expand our capacity for growth.

If a cycle provides an excess of the energy that is already built into us, that can make our lives harder. Things won't work in our favor for that cycle or the next if they are similar. This may not be what we want but it's coming to stay for a while. But we can do something about it to reduce the impact.

When we are in harmony, we know what to follow. We know what is coming and prepare accordingly. But most of us discredit the wisdom that comes from within, meeting it with disbelief as we chase external thoughts instead. We believe we are heading somewhere with our thoughts and logic, but in reality, we have taken no steps to improve.

We have an external information system of accumulated knowledge that we have sourced from books, people, news, internet, etc. However, we also have an internal information system. Do we even know that we have it? Well, we should.

The internal information is not from our head. To reach it, we must go beyond the surface and go much deeper. Reaching within is easy for some, and not so easy for others. In order to gain clarity in our search for inner wisdom, we seek and practice many forms of yoga, meditation, religion, and Zen to reach deeper connections. We instinctively know what it is. It is just a matter of finding a way in.

Many have died without having recognized the inherent wisdom housed in their body. They will need to learn it eventually with another body. Again, it's not about fairness or whether we like it or not. It's simply important to attend to our body's needs so that we can journey into the continuum.

As we learn about ourselves today, and in the course of a cycle of twelve years, hopefully we will become experts of our own physical, mental, emotional, and spiritual body.

To weather the storms of life, be sure to supply our organs with what they need to run a well-functioning body that will support us on our journey.

The unwise think that the good times will last forever and that this life is the only one they've got. So they mistreat themselves and others, not realizing that all of it will later come back to haunt them without fail. The wise, on the other hand, know to be good to themselves and others through both good times and bad. They have established a virtue account to help them grow, expand, and evolve.

My Observation and Investigative Results for 2021-2032

(Make a copy for each year to record observations, to learn, and to apply.)

Year:_____

The positive things that I noticed, and how I benefited:

The negatives things that I noticed, and how I benefited:

What was learned:

Through the help of inner guidance, how did I minimize the impact?

What did I to do turn a bad situation around?

What did I do to remedy my health issues?

What are the things that I noticed about my body system?

Learn and apply.

Chapter 8

More Things We Can Do to Improve

When There is Extreme Drought in the Kidney System

When our body is in drought condition, the body sends out chills or cold sensations. Our head and emotions only know to drink something warm like coffee (adding fire to the system), misinterpreting and misdirecting our body's need and further exacerbating the drought condition.

In reality, the problem is arising from excess warmth/heat in the body system that is tipping the body off balance. In other words, the cooling system is not working, due to insufficient Kidney energy to cool down the body. Therefore, it is essential that we supply our body with Kidney energy food so the other organ systems don't burn and melt down. Our logic and emotions cannot and will not understand the body's mechanism. Nevertheless, it is *our* responsibility as the owner of our body to know the difference and supply what's needed.

The following symptoms will disappear when either we supply the body with what it needs, or if we are lucky, it turns out to be just a condition passing through. The following list shows how each dominant organ type behaves, reacts, or signals differently under extreme dryness of the Kidneys.

Kidney

Mostly happy during this time.

Heart

- anxious/unstable
- back pain
- burning sensations
- (muscles, tendons, joints really on internal fire)
- charlie horse
- dry and stiff eyes
- excruciating pain when extreme, (torture-like stretching, pulling, "severing" of body parts)
- loss of hair
- tightness/dislocation of jaws
- frequent kidney stones
- lymph issues

- dry mouth, tight and sandy
- muscle weakness/pain
- restless sleep
- shivering
- mentally/physically/ emotionally sluggish
- skin tightness, itchiness, swelling
- teeth ache (lower jaw)
- thyroid trouble
- bubbles in urine
- strong odor from urine
- burning/pain sensation during urination
- feels off-balance/unsteady

Liver

- anxious
- back issues
- excess dry eyes
- joint pains
- kidney stones
- hot flashes
- nervousness
- withdrawn
- sluggish
- stomach dryness
- tooth problems/ ache/pain
- tension
- weakening of the muscles

Lung

- anxious
- back pains
- burning sensation of the muscles
- charlie horse
- choking sensation
- eyes dry, stiff, sensitive
- hot flashes
- jaw tightness
- joint discomfort
- kidney stone (rare)
- feels off-balance/unsteady
- restless sleep
- tightness of upper back ceiling of the mouth, film build up
- muscle tightness/weakness
- muscles feel fragile, breakable (soon turns numb, covering the symptoms)
- calcium build-up on the teeth and gum lines, aches/pains
- intense pressure/burning sensation on tooth
- itchy skin
- sluggish mental function
- burning sensation during urination
- bubbles in urine
- strong odor from urine

Stomach

- back pain
- burning sensation of the muscle
- charlie horse
- choking sensation
- dry and stiff eyes
- face appears smaller and darker
- gum ache/tightness
- hair loss
- graying of hair
- hot flashes
- jaw tightness/dislocation
- frequent kidney stones
- lymph issues
- thyroid issues
- aching of teeth

(Stomach, continued)

- mouth feels sandy, with white film buildup
- muscle aches/weakness/pain
- sluggish body
- itchy skin
- skin expansion
- shivering

- restless sleep
- bubbles in urine
- strong odor from urine
- burning/pain sensation during urination
- feels off-balanced/unsteady on feet
- tingling toes, fingers

How Do We Remedy the Extreme Drought in the Body System?

Provide Kidneys with extra amounts of what it needs for the following dominant organs.

Heart:

4–5 glasses of aloe vera juice (no sugar), or as needed

Liver:

1–2 glasses of aloe vera juice (no sugar)

Lung:

2–3 glasses of organic cranberry juice, or as needed

Stomach:

4–5 glasses of 100% cranberry juice (no sugar added) and aloe vera juice (no sugar added) combined to make 50/50 to drink daily, or as needed

What Beneficial Places Can I Go To With My Strong Organ Energies?

When extreme conditions/situations occur, our excess organ energy takes over our body. It has no consideration for the other organs that must all work together to survive. With the excessively strong organ taking over all the energies, the weaker organs, unable to support themselves and the system, soon begin to deteriorate and collapse.

Therefore, don't feed the strong organ. Instead, we must feed the weaker organs, supplying them with the foods they need. Otherwise, we won't be able to stand on our own and make it through our life's journey, in contrast to what our strong organ/s would have us believe.

A strong organ is tough to take, but when it has extreme excess energy, it is much tougher. It favors the wrong foods in order to match its current extreme condition, and rejects anything that might be beneficial and bring balance to the body. Just because it is powerful enough to dominate over other organs doesn't mean it has enough common sense to save itself. It will lead to self-destruction and take everything with it. So, we must be smart and be responsible owners of our body!

Go to places that will provide what's lacking in our body system. All we have to do is just be there and allow the land/location to heal us as it replenishes the missing energies in our body. However, there is a likelihood that our partner may not like the places we need to go simply because he/she may already have plenty of that energy in their system.

Strong Kidney-Kidney

Excess will break the balance of your body.

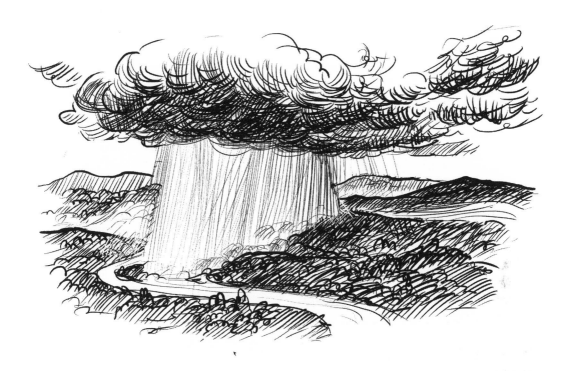

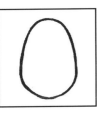

Kidney-Kidney

Too much Kidney energy will break the balance of the entire system. This creates a very damp condition in the body, making it susceptible to molds, viruses, and germs.

- Take in *triple* the amount of the foods from the recommended list.
- Avoid everything from the Kidney food list at all cost.

Where to go?

A weeklong vacation in Arizona (especially Grand Canyon and Sedona) will calm the body and dry it out rather quickly. Some may not consider it a proper vacation. However, for the strong Kidney body it's a very good vacation.

How will we know this? Finally, our body will begin to see more, have more room to breathe, and feel free with fewer busy thoughts.

Strong Heart-Heart

Excess will break the balance of your body.

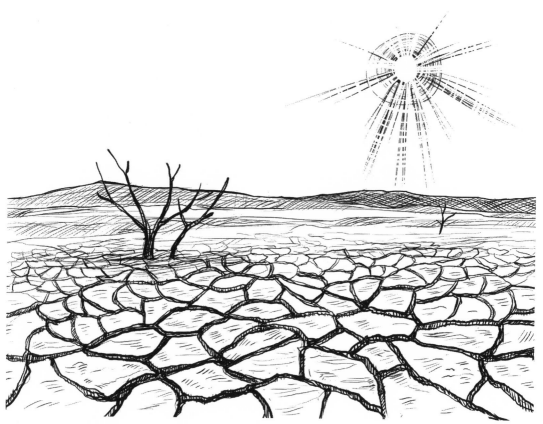

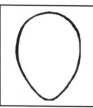

Heart-Heart

All airways tighten and increase blood pressure due to heat expansion within our body system. The extreme heat creates a fog in the system as well. Our body system will use all the available resources in our body, including the bone marrow.

- We must supply our body with what it needs if we want to continue to exist.
- Avoid everything under the Heart food list at all cost.

Where to go?

Take a trip to Alaska, Seattle, Mt. Rainier, Vancouver B.C., Ocean Shores, or do a full body soak in the healing mineral waters of Soap Lake, WA.

Strong Liver-Liver

Excess Liver will injure the Stomach and keep it from holding and supporting the excess Liver energy.

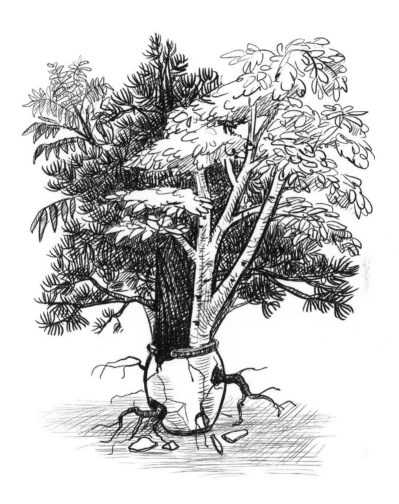

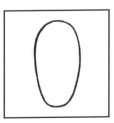

Liver-Liver

Where to go?

Take a trip to Arches National Park, Yosemite National Park, Mt. Rainier National Park, or Zion National Park, where there are many rocks. Palouse Prairie or any vast farm fields are also good places to visit.

How will we know that we've benefited from the trip?

We will experience freedom from confinement.

Strong Lung-Lung

Excess Lung energy overworks the Heart.

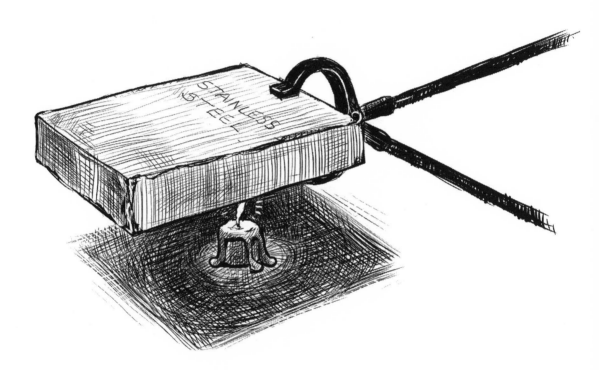

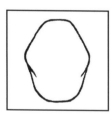

Lung-Lung

- Avoid everything from the Lung food list at all cost.
- Avoid bodies of water. It will weaken the Heart system.

Where to go?

Take a trip to Olympic National Park, Arches National Park, Great Smokey Mountains National Park, Mt. Baker National Park, or any deeply forested area. Or, do a full body soak in the healing mineral waters of Soap Lake, WA.

Strong Stomach-Stomach

Excess Stomach energy makes it extra difficult for the Kidney to function properly.

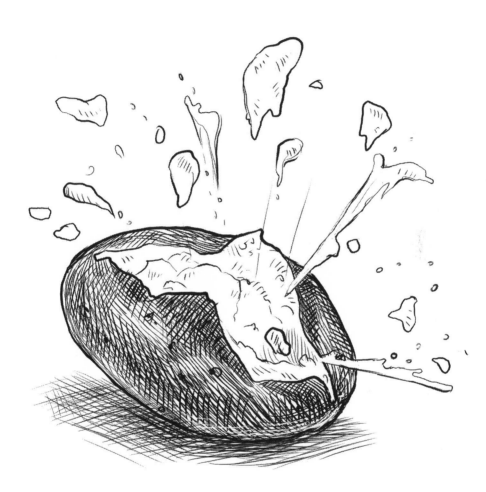

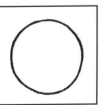

Stomach-Stomach

Where to go?

Spend time near a body of water, like lakes, rivers and oceans. Alaska and Mt. Baekdu are also good places to go. You can also go to Olympic National Park, Crater Lake, OR, or do a full body soak in the healing mineral waters of Soap Lake, WA.

How to Improve Health, Money, Dignity, and Longevity

Sometimes, we seem to be on a lucky streak when it comes to money, love, health, fame, power, dignity, and longevity. And sometimes, it seems like all those things disappear without a warning.

However, warning signs were given. We just didn't pay attention or we chose to neglect it. Perhaps it was because our organ system was ill-equipped to interpret the messages correctly and deliver them to us.

Our body sends out consistent communication on the changes within us and the outside world. To have the communication be clear, our body has to function properly.

What if a great opportunity to prosper arrives, but our body system is in too poor a condition to receive it, due to broken parts within that system? Until the broken parts are fixed, we will lose that opportunity to prosper.

Some of us pray to our God/gods to provide us with what we need. God/gods provides. However, we lose whatever that was and arrive at the same place of brokenness and need. Without true recognition of our condition, we will continue to do the same and be stuck in that same spot no matter how much we receive from our God/gods.

The universe is very fair and continually runs on cycles that provide each and every one the chance to succeed and prosper. If someone seems to have taken more than their share of things, it's not their fault. They simply made it so that they had greater capacity to hold more than what they needed. Rather, it is our fault for not repairing our system so it can hold the share that was given to us.

If money is what we want, there's still plenty to go around after we fix our broken system.

If love is what we want, support the organ that handles it. There are so many wonderful people looking to share their love with others. It will be different for each person.

If power is what we want, support the organ that handles it. There are unlimited resources out there, but they must be used wisely. It will be different for each person.

If dignity is what we want, support that organ which handles it. It will be different for each person.

If fame is what we want, support that organ which handles it. It will be different for each person.

If longevity is what we want, follow nature's way to support our body with slow/deep breathing and reduced sexual activity. One sexual event diminishes our finite resource of most precious life energy and makes us grow older more quickly. This applies to all who are looking for a way to live longer with mental clarity.

Take extra of these food items for your dominant organ/s. However, make sure to fill any holes in your system first. Things will improve.

Be sure to stay within all other organs' capacity.

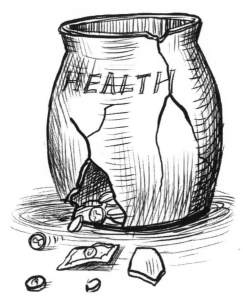

Health: Good health will naturally bring in money, love, power, and fame.

<u>**For Strong Kidney**</u>: bitter foods, bell flower root, lamb, coffee, green tea, chocolate, dandelions, corn, ginseng, codonopsis

<u>**For Strong Heart**</u>: beef, fish, aloe vera juice, almond, mint, pepper, gingko, pine nuts, hot spice

<u>**For Strong Liver**</u>: sweet tasting foods, sweet potato, sweet rice, honey, royal jelly, propolis, ginseng

<u>**For Strong Lungs**</u>: greens, beans, chicken, grapes, apples, all nuts (except almonds and pine nuts), ginseng

<u>**For Strong Stomach**</u>: greens, greens, greens, seaweed, cranberries, black tea, bone broth soup, berry tea, pork, sea cucumber

✵ Avoid sleeping and living in a geopathic stress zone.

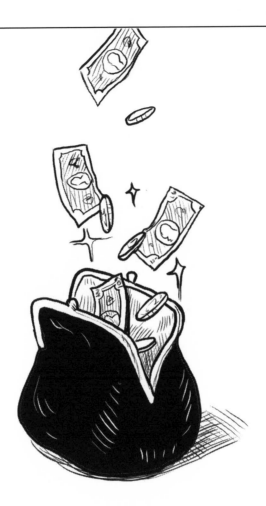

Money: To improve.

For Strong Kidney: bitter foods, lamb, coffee, green tea, chocolate, dandelions, corn, ginseng, bell flower root, codonopsis

For Strong Heart: beef, fish, aloe vera juice, almond, mint, pepper, hot spice

For Strong Liver: sweet tasting foods, sweet potato, sweet rice, honey, royal jelly, ginseng

For Strong Lungs: greens, beans, chicken, grapes, apples, all nuts (except almonds and pine nuts)

For Strong Stomach: greens, greens, greens, seaweed, pork, cranberries, black tea, bone broth soup, berry tea

✱ Avoid sleeping and living in a geopathic stress zone.

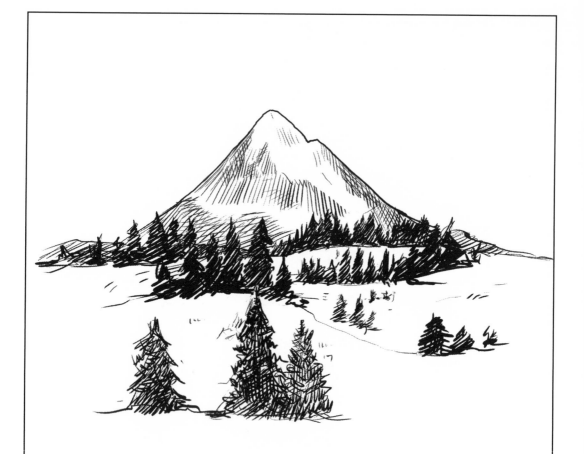

Dignity: Increase intake.

<u>For Strong Kidney</u>: lots of sweets, chocolate, lamb, turkey, root vegetables, ginseng, royal jelly

<u>For Strong Heart</u>: lots of beef, fish, aloe vera juice, cranberry, cucumber, mushroom, pork, cherries

<u>For Strong Liver</u>: beef, fish, some sweets, mint, pepper, hot spice

<u>For Strong Lungs</u>: lamb, coffee, green tea, chocolate, turkey, corn, greens

<u>For Strong Stomach</u>: greens, cranberry juice, beans, chicken, pork, apple, grapes

✳ Avoid sleeping and living in a geopathic stress zone.

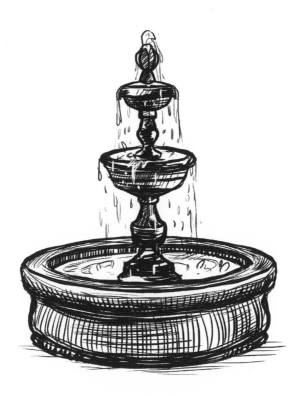

Longevity: What to do and what not to do.

We must be not too happy, not too sad, not so angry, and not so depressed. And do natural breathing practices, follow nature's way of supporting our body system, eat what our body needs, chew our food well before swallowing, and reduce sexual activities.

Sex gives us great excitement, joy, connection, togetherness, contentment, and sometimes the heavenly feeling of wholeness. The heavenly feeling of wholeness stems from our longing to connect. However, there are other ways to become whole and be connected to our higher self. One sexual event will take away the most precious life energy from our reservoir more than any other act, aging us quickly and reducing our mental sharpness. When we are young, we don't care about that because it feels like this life energy is going to be there forever always. However, the wise learn to control their sexual appetite. They know that too much could haunt them later in life. Therefore, the wise understand and apply the virtue of temperance.

❋ Avoid sleeping and living in a geopathic stress zone.

As we take in these food items, we will begin to see the changes that take place in us physically, mentally, emotionally, and spiritually.

Everything is processed so effortlessly and all the benefits of these changes are so fully utilized, that the changes simply slide into our daily habits and we don't notice the changes as much as we should. Even without us acknowledging it, we live better with a better functioning body that no longer demands our attention with its pain and discomfort. This is natural, and the way it should be for a well-functioning body.

In contrast, observant outsiders who see us only occasionally will recognize the changes and let us know that something has shifted and improved in us.

However, if we live in the present moment, keenly paying attention with an observant, investigative, and fair mind, we will fully recognize the changes as they occur, and know the truth.

Whereas we may be slow to notice the changes, the dominant organ functions on the other hand will know immediately the changes that are occurring. Fearful of losing its dominance, it will do anything to stop us from continuing to improve our whole body system and harmonize our energies. It will begin to fill our thoughts with negativity and false information, laying out various reasons why we shouldn't continue, and why it's all a worthless pursuit, etc. It will work to influence our thoughts continuously, and create as much doubt as possible in the hopes that we give up. By this way, it works to remain the dominant organ in our body system.

We never think to know what our particular organ functions are capable of. Can our organ functions actually hijack our thoughts and make us believe that their thoughts are our thoughts, and their choices our choices?

Let's reflect and observe. We will take an example that all of us can relate to. Let's say that we remember to nurture our body by eating and drinking things that are beneficial for us. So we march into the kitchen with this intention and open the refrigerator door. But for some reason, we stare blankly into the refrigerator, suddenly forgetting why we are there. Our mind blank, we pick an item or two that our dominant organ likes and close the refrigerator door. Is this a fluke, or did the dominant-organ function or something else influence us?

Let's assume it is the organ function that is influencing us. It doesn't know right from wrong, or what is beneficial or harmful. It simply carries out its function on a continuing basis. Using clever thought tricks, it manipulates us into thinking that we made these decisions ourselves, without the organ's influence. And when something bad happens, it doesn't take responsibility for the situation. It will be up to us to clean up after its mess and pay for any damages now and into the future.

This is a great ride for the dominant organ. It holds no responsibility for what it does, and it never pays the price for any of its actions. Why would the dominant organ give this up? It won't, and it will continue to play this game as long as we allow it to deceive us, and we remain ignorant of our rights and responsibilities. The dominant organ is only carrying out its natural function, and it will continue to keep going until we step in to correct it. So, don't blame them. Rather, we should ask ourselves, "Is this what I want for my life?"

What do we do with mere functions that are part of us?

The dominant organ doesn't know that it needs the other organs for it to thrive. Nor can we expect it to have consideration for any of the related organ systems that can help it to function better. This capacity of thought is not part of its function. This capacity to see and care for the whole body is given to us. But instead of exercising this given capacity ourselves, why do we assume and expect these mere functions to provide for us and take care of us when such a program was never installed into them? Maybe this is where much of our frustration arises from, and we have not come to realize it yet.

Once our organs are somewhat harmonized, we'll be able to see ourselves in a broader light, and be able to do more than before.

How do I know that I am getting there?

When we reach a somewhat harmonized body structure, we will gain clarity and a broader perspective on things that before we weren't quite able to see in their fullness, such as kindness, fairness, and compassion. And, because we feel much more content with a harmonized internal body structure, we'll be able to be less judgmental of ourselves and others. Be present to realize these things and know our rights and responsibilities. We can teach, nurture, and grow our organ functions, allowing them to mature into a noble human being to the fullest extent possible. We do this because, ultimately, it is our responsibility.

However, if we have not reached a certain level of harmonized state, we won't be able to accomplish this. There will be much negativity, resistance, and frequent hijacking of our thoughts by our organ functions. Be sure to acknowledge it when it happens.

To keep our life from spinning continuously, and to allow us to make certain changes to ourselves, we must continue to meet a certain level of harmonization in our organ body structure. And if we want to expedite this process of freeing ourselves from stress and agony, building up of a virtue account is recommended.

Why Do I Get Weird Dreams?

We sometimes get good dreams and sometimes terrible dreams even when we tell ourselves to dream better.

Dreams represent what is going on with our body system.

Some dreams are divine.
Some dreams are pleasant.
Some dreams predict what is to come.
Some dreams are terribly frightening.
Some dreams are horrific nightmares.
Some dreams show someone/something chasing us.

It is all depends on the condition of our body.

For example, when our body is in an optimal/wholesome condition, our dreams are positive and courageous, where everything seems to be in reach. There is no one chasing us, nor are we running away from anything. Without any hesitation, we stand, fight, and win, or avoid the fight altogether.

When our body condition is poor, in our dreams we are either backing down, are uncertain, confused, fearful, or chasing/running as a victim.

To change the bad dreams to something better, we must first fill the missing gaps within our body system and avoid going to bed on a full stomach. When we reach the point of having mended all the gaps, we will finally understand how important it is to take care of our body to get to where we want to go. **Please let us know when you reach this point so that it can benefit others on their journey.**

How Are Wifi and New Technology Affecting My Overall Health?

Wifi, smartphones, wireless routers, and cell towers are external energies that influence our body system. These modern technologies provide us with a great deal of convenience, entertainment and information, allowing us to do amazing things that weren't possible before.

However, without the careful use of this technology and the use of protective shielding devices to counter the damage done to our bodies, we will pay dearly with our health. Some people experience great suffering on a daily basis from the effects of these modern technologies. And some are aware of the dangers while some remain completely unaware. No matter how great or small our awareness of the dangers, this technology affects us all without exception.

Some who are less sensitive to the technology are the Stomach and Stomach-Heart types. It just means they are slow to acknowledge the damage and are in no way exempt from it. By the time the Stomach and Stomach-Heart come to realize the problem, it is often too late. Without exception, everyone's health is at stake, damaging us physically, emotionally, financially, and spiritually.

Without its careful use and the use of protective devices to lessen the bodily damage, these modern devices will end up altering the quality of our lives and our longevity without us realizing it. The biggest problem is that there is no medicine that can fix the damage done by them.

Breathing Meditation

We breathe every day, every hour, and every second of our day. Breathing is very basic to our survival. We have the right to breathe as much as we need and best of all, it's free.

Then what's so special about breathing? Well, because somewhere along the line, we forgot how to deeply breathe into our roots and connect. Our lives are busy, demanding our full presence on a continual basis. We are often chasing hectic schedules and life events that leave us trying to catch our breath. So, we've forgotten how to breathe deeply. We forgot about its power to calm the body and the mind, even when we are gripped by our daily demands. Carve out a time and find a quiet place to practice deep breathing until you are able to do it anywhere and anytime.

Take time to focus on your breathing.

You will notice that your mental chatter is going on randomly. Don't be alarmed by it. Just let it be. It's nothing special. It's just a function that does it whether we are aware of it or not.

If this is your first time doing a breathing practice, let's start with Lung Breathing.

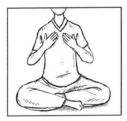 *Palms to chest*   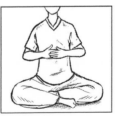 *Palms to stomach*

Lung Breathing

1. This should be done on an empty stomach, or 1 hour after a meal.
2. You can sit, stand, or lie down to straighten your back.

3. Rest both palms on the chest. (*See illustration on previous page.*)
4. Exhale and inhale through the mouth and nose, breathing naturally without forcing more air into the lungs.
5. Focus on exhaling all the way out. Let the air come through your mouth and nostrils as naturally as possible. Don't force more air into your lungs.
6. After 5–10 mins of doing this, you will notice that your breathing is much more calm and less bothered by mental chatters.
7. Continue to do this for the next 5–6 days, for 20 minutes at a time.
8. From this state, our expansion of knowing will occur, getting a glimpse of realization and knowing here and there. By practicing deep breathing daily, you will have less stress.
9. Once the lung is done, it goes down to the stomach automatically.
10. Rest palms on the stomach area. (*See illustration on previous page.*)
11. Breathe through the mouth and nostrils.
12. Exhale any toxins in the stomach area, exhaling all the way.
13. Inhale only what the body requires, but exhale to push out a bit more.
14. You may become drowsy and fall asleep. That's okay.
15. Continue until your breathing takes you to the lower abdomen.
16. Take a walk after each breathing exercise.

Lower Abdomen Breathing

1. Exhale, seeing yourself exhaling out all the toxins in your system. As you do this, your body will want to breathe in. Allow only to its capacity.
2. Focus only on exhaling out all the way until the body wants to inhale.
3. Stay with your breath. As you do this, you will realize that your muscles and joints are beginning to relax with your breathing.
4. Rest both palms on navel (*see illustration "Palms to low abdomen."*)
5. Still focus on the exhale, not the inhale.
6. As you draw out your exhale, your body will automatically hold the breath until it wants to inhale. Follow with that.
7. Follow your inhale, taking in air until it reaches capacity and the body is ready to exhale. Follow that.
8. When you do this, there is no forced breathing to create problems for you.
9. Push more on exhaling all the way out, imagining all the toxins leaving your body through your breath.
10. Once the toxins are out, your body will breathe automatically on its own.
11. Follow with natural breathing.

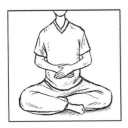

Palms to low abdomen

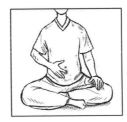

Finger to dahn-jun

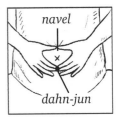

Focus on dahn-jun

Dahn-jun Breathing

1. Put a finger on the dahn-jun below the navel and focus on it, lightly pressing as you exhale (*see illustration "Finger to dahn-jun."*)
2. Never be greedy in the inhale, trying to force in extra air. Just follow the body's natural capacity.
3. Soon you will find your body breathing like a baby.
4. Let it happen, with no interference from you.
5. You are where the dahn-jun is, the place where children breathe into normally, deeply and peacefully.
6. You just breathe, only focusing on dahn-jun. If there is mental chatter going on, let it be. That's its function. You only focus on the dahn-jun.
7. This is a place of peace. From here you will know and have a glimpse of realization. There will be an expansion of energy and knowing.
8. After a good breathing practice, do some light exercise or take 10–30 minute walk.
9. By doing this breathing exercise daily, you will experience many realizations and have less stress from daily activities.

**See Saving Me First 2, p. 200–201 for postures if you want to continue to the next level. However, remember to never exceed your body's natural capacity. Never try to force increase in breathing intervals.

Twice Prospered, Twice Broken, and a Third Chance

This story is about an organ-driven auto-pilot program that was running a certain woman's life. However, she changed her life around by making some adjustments to her food intake and adding one new habit.

I had known this woman for a long time. She would make money left and right for a while and then she would go broke. Several years later, again she would make money left and right, accumulating assets. Two years before she was to lose everything again, I visited her to find a way to warn her that she was going to lose everything and be very poor once more.

I advised her to prepare herself in the next two years for the looming disaster. She wouldn't listen. At that moment, she couldn't imagine it happening. Yes, she had experienced it before, but she felt that she was much smarter now. She wouldn't let it happen twice.

Still, I explained further that a hole in her body system would begin to widen, becoming a giant hole through which she would lose all her fortune. If she was going to lose it anyway, why not make donations to a good cause? That good deed would return to her as a virtue account that would help her when she needed it. She didn't like what I had to say.

Two years later, she found herself in court when a trusted friend had taken off after borrowing over two million dollars from her. The downward spiral continued until she was completely broke with a mountain of debts. And yet, she was confident that she would make it through because she had done it before. She was banking on that. However, she had never been that broke before and no matter what she tried, she sank deeper into debt.

Several years later, she came to me and wanted to know what she could do to come back up. I told her that wasn't my area of expertise. However, I could help her patch that hole in her body system that had led her to this point. She wanted a miracle. I told her that if in this life she managed to block the hole inside of her, that would be a miracle in itself. Otherwise, she would continue to go up and down on her crazy endless cycles. The only way to stop this was for her to realize and do something about it.

She was reaching her 60s and so didn't have much time left to ride the up cycle again. And she needed to come up again as she didn't have any savings for her retirement and was facing numerous debts she couldn't pay. She considered filing for bankruptcy but chose not to. She wanted to climb back up and leave something for her children and grandkids. She wondered why she couldn't live like other people.

With no other options before her, she decided to fill the holes in her body system and do donations as I had suggested before. She had lost everything so with nothing to lose, she would try this new method of fixing herself.

She was too ashamed to ask others for help. She came to me knowing that I had no money to give her, and that I was the only one she could trust to keep her shameful situation a secret. She also knew that I never asked for anything from her or other people, and lived very content and happy despite not having a lot of money. If possible, she wanted some of that contentment and peace too.

In order to get her started on her new beginning, I borrowed funds from my friend and asked the woman's daughter to help any way she could to help start a new business. Her daughter created a minus account for her to use as she needed and to pay back whenever she could. Her outlook was good and she moved ahead with her new business.

As usual, she began making money. She paid her debts to me and her daughter in two years. All her other debts were paid in full three years after that. Completely free from her debts, she thanked me for the help.

She promised to donate a certain amount every year to food banks, religious groups, hunger funds, etc. no matter what. She did this willingly, saying this was the least she could do.

Then she slowed down. Greed was creeping in as she thought about how she could leave more money to her grandkids if she didn't donate so much. She got excited over the thought of accumulating money.

She informed me that she wouldn't be donating like before. I told her no problem. That was her decision to make. However, she needed to understand that the different supports that she and her family had been receiving would no longer be available from that point on. She said she was okay with that. She chose not to know what that meant, and she chose not to remember the promises that she had made before. The greedy and ignorant mind had no integrity or shame. It wanted to believe that her prosperity was all due to her good luck and didn't want to share the wealth with others.

Though it was a foolish decision on her part, I didn't try to convince her otherwise. She needed to learn it for herself. It was a process she had to go through to reach the next step. And that was only if she was awake and actually chose to take the next step.

Soon, she noticed that the extra income she was counting on wasn't coming in. No matter how she calculated, there was no extra money. After many months of doing this, she started to get angry at the situation. She prayed but it didn't turn out as she hoped. From that point on, her outlook became very negative.

She had made a choice, and she would live with it. Once the greedy mind took over, she became a different person. Her greed was in charge now. This was a process of growing. It was a process of learning to choose how she wanted to live her life. This was her decision to make, not mine.

After two years had passed, she finally got in touch with her conscience and realized that she had to change her stupid greedy mind and come back to reality. She decided to resume with her donations. This was one of the wisest decisions that she had made for herself, for her own sake. The money in her possession wasn't hers or her sons' in the first place. Even if she tried to keep it, it would slip away from her and her sons anyway.

At the beginning, what the greedy mind wanted seemed like the smart thing to do. But in reality, it was really foolish because her prosperity included someone else's share. To try to keep it would be stealing and cheating from those who helped her to get there. The donations were a sign of her appreciation for that help and she in return were helping others in need. That's how it was designed.

After reflecting on various parts of herself, she had a realization and decided to continue with her donations to those less fortunate. She was able to come to this self-benefiting realization because she had been taking good care of her body system. Had she not done so and neglected her body, she would have gone the other way, believing that she had made the right choice as she returned to being broke, both financially and physically in her organ systems.

For how long would she be able to function from this new place of wisdom? As long as she took good care of her body, and maintained the harmony of her organ systems to some degree, she would be able to continue making wise choices.

I was glad for her. If she hadn't done this, she would have been a servant to her greed. The greedy mind only knows greed and nothing else. It doesn't know how the universe works and what is the right thing to do. Had she kept following her greed, she wouldn't have known that her greedy mind was cheating her of this deeper greater knowledge.

Sharing our wealth with others, along with good deeds/charity work, guarantees our continued survival and maintaining of the wealth we have now and in the future.

Ten years later, she is healthier than ever before and still running the business she had started when she hit rock bottom for the second time, buried in debt. Now, her wealth has grown to three houses and several bank accounts.

It's important to first fill the holes in our body system. Next, creating a virtue account by doing good deeds for others in need can help us now, or on a future rainy day. It can even benefit our loved ones into their future. The benefits from good deeds are beyond what we imagine. The return on good deeds and charitable donations pays handsomely. In my experience, no other investment gives this much in return.

Try to create a virtue account for yourself and be wise. You'll get to live life with less stress and agony. To fill your virtue account is to create abundant blessings for yourself.

Chapter 9

The Cycle of Seasons

The Cycle of Energies
That Affects Our Health, Money, Fame, Power, Dignity, and Longevity

There are times when it feels like everything lines up when it comes to health, money, love, fame, power, dignity, and longevity.

And there are times when everything goes up in smoke and feels like nothing is going right. It all comes with the changing seasons and it all goes with the shifting cycles.

We have a built-in warning system to alert us of the changes, but we often choose not to respect or honor this internal warning, which is rooted in our inner wisdom. It knows what is happening to us at all times. But instead, we choose to listen to some group or individual to tell us what to do and what is good for us. How do they know when they don't listen to, or understand, their own body system? But we follow them anyway because they promise to take away the burden of self-care. We love it that we don't have to be responsible for taking care of ourselves anymore. But does this burden actually disappear?

From our organs' operative point of view, our body systems are very complicated and hard to logically figure out. It is this dependence on logic that relinquishes our self-care to someone else.

When we neglect parts of ourselves, someone or something may be directly benefiting from that neglect. And we allow others to make decisions for us and direct our lives. That's okay if that's what we have chosen.

And having someone else to deal with our health issues sounds like a great thing, even if the information they have isn't always correct, or they actually have no idea and are experimenting on us.

But who ultimately suffers as a direct result of this? We do. We tend to overlook the signals coming from our own body and choose to neglect it. We suffer as a consequence because it's our body that we are neglecting. Why are we looking to someone else to manage our body for even the smallest discomfort? We're already equipped with so much knowledge within our manual. If we must look to others, let's find the expert of experts when it comes to our body.

The $995 Answer

About 20 years ago, Sun Doh master Paul and I attended a two-day lecture/workshop that cost us $995 each. We thought it was overpriced but we attended anyway, despite not having a lot of money back then. We just charged it on our credit card.

After the first day of lecture, we very much regretted our decision to attend. There was nothing worthwhile for us in the lecture. The second day, however, was different. Something that the speaker said woke us up. He said that most poor people (financially insecure) tend to ask their neighbors, friends, colleagues or family members for advice on tax matters, finances and investments.

"What made you think to ask them these questions?" he asked the audience.

That startled us, because we were doing that. We assumed that the people we asked knew more than us. However, we really didn't get anything out of it by asking any of our friends, family, and acquaintances. We still carried the question in us.

"Do you know why you are still in the situation you are in?" he asked.

Everyone wanted to know the secret, the $995 answer.

"You are too cheap to find the expert of experts to help you move forward with your dreams." he told us.

We had met many "qualified" experts, or those who claimed to be experts. However, we still found ourselves stuck in the same place, running madly but going nowhere like a hamster in its wheel.

We never thought that we were cheap. We worked hard and were very serious about working toward our goals, but didn't know how to go about achieving them.

After the lecture, the speaker was passing by and greeted us with a smile. So I ventured a question. "Where do I even begin to look for those experts? There are so many of them. How will I know the right one?"

He gave us his business card and said, "Call me tomorrow."

He told us to get out of the "poor comfort zone" that we were in. To move ourselves into the next phase of our lives, we had to stop operating from that mindset.

This was common sense, but the way he had delivered the message and the tools he had provided allowed us to make things happen. We followed his advice and maintained the teams that were established back then, utilizing the tools he provided. For a lecture, that was the most well spent $995.

In the end, we saved a great deal of time, money, and stress when we found the expert of experts to give us the right answers.

So, when it comes to our body, don't find an unqualified person for our body's need just to have emotional support. Find the expert of experts who knows exactly what we can do to keep us well.

Secrets of the Body

Our body system is not a simple one. It is a giant meticulous system, consisting of 365 meridian stations designed to connect to the universe and to flow harmoniously with it. And this system comes with the manual already attached.

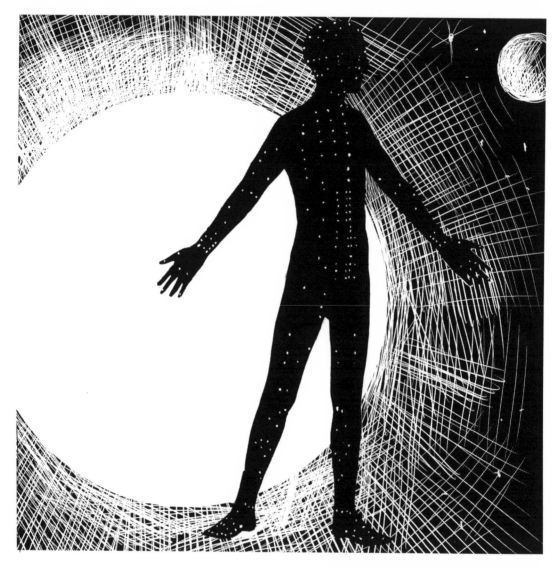

The connection is not only for humans but for all living and non-living beings.

The energy lights up each station as it arrives at certain times of the day. If one of the stations is out of order, its likely that no signal will be transmitted to us.

If one of the system's stations goes out, the system creates an alternate route to make a connection until the station can be fixed. Once repaired, the system returns to its original route.

From time to time, all 365 meridian stations would light up at once when all systems are harmonized. At that point, we are fully connected to the universe, completely awed by what we experience and the knowledge we attain. This lighting up of all stations occurs at different times for different body structures.

This system is both divine and amazingly complicated, running to the precise minute, hour, day, month, year, decade and even century. It is our responsibility to do regular maintenance when it gives us the signal.

To Access the Manual
Within Us...

To access the manual within us,
there's one requirement.
It is the desire to know and understand who we are.

To understand in depth, continue inward inquiry/koan.*
Do not expect anything. Only the solid awareness.
When we are able to connect with solid awareness for
72 hours, either through meditative solitude or
our normal daily life,

the ultimate answer will reveal itself.

All questions and mysteries of life will disappear with the
full understanding of the greater life itself.

If this is the true experience, we don't have to worry or try
to make something up.
We can directly access the Ultimate Manual within us every
moment, effortlessly.

*Koan: a riddle Zen Buddhists use during meditation to
help them unravel greater truths about themselves and the
world.

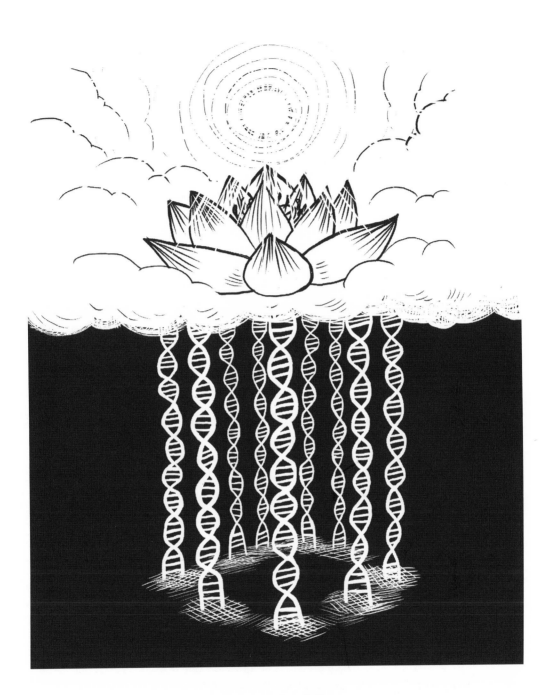

Unseen Ladders

Although it cannot be seen through our physical eyes, we are all part of this divine nature. When we have strong Will and certain virtue accounts in place, we can finally be reunited.

Virtue Account

For the givers, whatever the gift may be, it must be given without condition and without expecting anything in return. It must be given freely without doubt, grumbling, or calculation of any kind. Once given, we let it go, and must not cling to the idea of how great and kind we are, or wish to be recognized for the deed. That's the ego talking. We give and let go. We have already received a blessing in the act itself. And we do our giving as discreetly as possible, without fanfare. This way of giving guarantees the highest return possible for the virtue account.

For the receivers, whatever gift is received, no matter how humble, we receive with sincere appreciation of that gift. There is no judging or weighing of that gift. By accepting the gifts with whole sincerity, we are allowing the other person to fill their virtue account as we fill our own. We are in essence, blessing each other in the exchange.

One is everything.
Everything is One.
Therefore, all things are we, us, ours,
and ourselves.

Summary of the Cycles

As we can see and experience from the cycles of life, nothing stays forever. It gives no preference for the poor, rich, woman, or man. It doesn't care where we live, or what race we are, or what religion we believe or not believe in. None of it really matters. All the cycles come and go, affecting all of us. This especially matters to those stuck in the wheel of suffering. Some of us want to be free of the suffering but don't know how to get out. To be free, supply what the organs need to run a body that is balanced and well-functioning. With a healthy body, we will gain the strength to see the problems that hold us down and take ourselves out of our suffering.

Some cycle years prove to be good for one group while not so good for another, and vice versa. This cycle will continue on and the exact combination of cycles will meet up every 60 years. The universe runs on this cycle and gives everyone a fair chance to grow whether we know it or not.

The energies of the universe change all the time, as does our body system. The only things that do not change with the flow are our fixed thought patterns. That's not nature's way. However, some of us insist on continually being stuck, caught in the wheel of suffering. By adjusting our body system, we give ourselves a better chance of waking up from our delusions and free ourselves from the wheel of endless suffering.

Let's wake up.

Let's live with full awareness *right now*, not clinging to even a single thought, and be well connected to our inner true self. And let's unlock the chains of suffering and live our lives to the fullest.

Wishing you and all of us a great and fruitful journey!

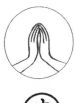

Notes

Made in the USA
Monee, IL
18 October 2020

44964685R00132